FOGSI EEBR 2025

Ethical Evidence-Based Recommendations

Hypertensive Disorders of Pregnancy

Disclaimer

This Ethical Evidence-Based Recommendation (EEBR) document is drafted following a consensus between esteemed FOGSI experts and stakeholders and are based on the scientific evidence available at the time of preparation.

EEBRs should be used for information and educational purposes. They do not replace the need for application of clinical judgment to each individual presentation, or variations based on individual patient and resource setting.

Furthermore, EEBRs do not constitute or imply the endorsement of any of the included technologies, therapies, or techniques by FOGSI.

FOGSI EEBR 2025

Ethical Evidence-Based Recommendations

Hypertensive Disorders of Pregnancy

Editor-in-Chief

Sunita Tandulwadkar
MD (Obs and Gyne) FICS (Gyne-Endoscopy) FICOG
President, FOGSI (2025–2026)
Gynecological Endoscopist and ART & IVF Specialist
Head, Department of Obstetrics and Gynecology
Chief, IVF & Endoscopy Center, Ruby Hall Clinic, Pune
Founder and Medical Director, Solo Clinic IVF—A Center for Excellence in Infertility and Endoscopy, Pune
Founder and Medical Director, Solo Stem Cells—A Stem Cell Research and Application Center, Pune
Founder and Director, Alive Regenerative Wellness, Pune, Maharashtra, India

Editors

Ameya C Purandare
MD DNB DGO DGP FCPS FICOG MNAMS
Consultant
Department of Obstetrics and Gynecology
Purandare Hospital, KJ Somaiya Medical College, Sir HN Reliance Hospital
Mumbai, Maharashtra, India

Palaniappan Narayanan
DNB FICOG FICS
Professor and Head
Department of Obstetrics and Gynecology
Sri Ramachandra Medical College
Chennai, Tamil Nadu, India

Experts

Suchitra Pandit
MD DNB MRCOG FRCOG FICOG DFP BPharm MNAMS
Senior Consultant
Department of Obstetrics and Gynecology
Surya Group of Hospitals
Mumbai, Maharashtra, India

Jayam Kannan
MD DGO
Director
Garbba Rakshambigai Fertility Center, Chennai
Emeritus Professor
Department of High-risk Obstetrics and Infertility
The Tamil Nadu Dr MGR Medical University
Chennai, Tamil Nadu, India

Convener

Pooja Lodha
DNB (Obs and Gyne)
Fellow, Fetal Medicine, FOGSI-FMF UK Certified
Lead Consultant
Department of Fetal Medicine
Ruby Hall Clinic and Bharati Vidyapeeth University and Hospital, Pune
Director, Kangaroo Cradle, Fetal Care Centre
Pune, Maharashtra, India

JAYPEE BROTHERS MEDICAL PUBLISHERS
The Health Sciences Publisher
New Delhi | London

Jaypee Brothers Medical Publishers (P) Ltd

Headquarters
Jaypee Brothers Medical Publishers (P) Ltd
EMCA House, 23/23-B
Ansari Road, Daryaganj
New Delhi 110 002, India
Landline: +91-11-23272143, +91-11-23272703
+91-11-23282021, +91-11-23245672
Email: jaypee@jaypeebrothers.com

Corporate Office
Jaypee Brothers Medical Publishers (P) Ltd
4838/24, Ansari Road, Daryaganj
New Delhi 110 002, India
Phone: +91-11-43574357
Fax: +91-11-43574314
Email: jaypee@jaypeebrothers.com

Overseas Office
JP Medical Ltd.
83, Victoria Street, London
SW1H 0HW (UK)
Phone: +44 20 3170 8910
Fax: +44 (0)20 3008 6180
Email: info@jpmedpub.com

Website: www.jaypeebrothers.com
Website: www.jaypeedigital.com

Inquiries for bulk sales may be solicited at: jaypee@jaypeebrothers.com

FOGSI EEBR 2025—Ethical Evidence-Based Recommendations: Hypertensive Disorders of Pregnancy

First Edition: **2025**

ISBN: 978-93-6616-153-2

Printed in India

Contributors

Abha Rani Sinha MS DGO FICOG
Principal-cum-Professor
Department of Obstetrics and Gynecology
Sri Krishna Medical College
Muzaffarpur, Bihar, India

Ameya C Purandare
MD DNB DGO DGP FCPS FICOG MNAMS
Senior Consultant
Department of Obstetrics and Gynecology
Purandare Hospital, KJ Somaiya Medical College, Sir HN Reliance Hospital
Mumbai, Maharashtra, India

Ashish Varma
MBBS MS FMAS DMAS FICRS FIVF
Assistant Professor
Department of Obsterics and Gynaecology
Narendra Modi Medical College
Sheth LG Hospital
Ahmedabad, Gujarat, India

Brihathi Pranavi Dasari
MBBS MS DNB
Senior Resident
Department of Obstetrics and Gynecology
Kasturba Medical College
Manipal, Karnataka, India

Deepali Kapote MS DGO FCPS FICOG
Additional Professor
Department of Obstetrics and Gynecology
Lokmanya Tilak Medical College and Hospital, Sion
Consultant
Jupiter Hospital
Thane West, Maharashtra, India

Hemant Mehta MD DA MCPS
Chair, Anesthesia and Pain Management
All Reliance Foundation Healthcare Initiatives
Department of Anesthesia and Pain Management
Sir HN Reliance Foundation Hospital
Mumbai, Maharashtra, India

Jayam Kannan MD DGO
Director
Garbba Rakshambigai Fertility Center
Chennai
Emeritus Professor
Department of High-risk Obstetrics and Infertility
The Tamil Nadu Dr MGR Medical University
Chennai, Tamil Nadu, India

K Aparna Sharma
MD DNB FICOG MNAMS Masters in Fetal Medicine
Professor
Department of Obstetrics and Gynecology
All India Institute of Medical Sciences
New Delhi, India

Komal N Chavan
MD DNB MNAMS FCPS DGO FICOG
Senior Consultant, Unit Chief
Department of Obstetrics and Gynecology
VN Desai Hospital
Mumbai, Maharashtra, India

Manju Lata Verma
MD PDCC (Fetal Medicine)
Additional Professor
Department of Obstetrics and Gynecology
King George's Medical University
Lucknow, Uttar Pradesh, India

Mitra Saxena
MD DNB FICMCH FICOG DIP (Endoscopy, Kiel)
Director and Head
Department of Obstetrics and Gynecology
Shri Ashwini Saxena
Rewari, Haryana, India

Munjal Pandya
MS (Obs and Gyne) FICOG DMIS
Associate Professor
Department of Obstetrics and Gynecology
Narendra Modi Medical College
Ahmedabad, Gujarat, India

Neena Malhotra
MD DNB FRCOG FAMS FICOG
Professor and Head
Department of Obstetrics and Gynecology
All India Institute of Medical Sciences
New Delhi, India

Palaniappan Narayanan
DNB FICOG FICS
Professor and Head
Department of Obstetrics and Gynecology
Sri Ramachandra Medical College
Chennai, Tamil Nadu, India

Parikshit Tank
MD DNB DGO DFP MNAMS FICOG FRCOG
Senior Consultant
Department of Obstetrics and Gynecology
Ashwini Maternity and Surgical Hospital, Jupiter Hospital
Mumbai, Maharashtra, India
Honorary Professor
Department of Assisted Reproduction
Pacific Medical College and Hospital
Udaipur, Rajasthan, India
Treasurer, Federation of Obstetrics and Gynecological Societies of India (FOGSI), 2021–2024
Joint Secretary, FOGSI, 2012
Joint Treasurer, FOGSI, 2018–2020
Chairperson, Safe Motherhood
FOGSI, 2014–2017

Prakash K Mehta
MD DGO DNB Diploma Medical Law
Professor and Head
Department of Obstetrics and Gynecology
Chief
Department of Maternal Fetal Medicine
Bhagwan Mahaveer Jain Hospital
Bengaluru, Karnataka, India

Rajasri G Yaliwal
MBBS MS (Obs and Gyne) FICOG
Professor and Unit Chief
Department of Obstetrics and Gynecology
BLDE(DU) Shri BM Patil Medical College Hospital and Research Centre
Vijayapura, Karnataka, India

Ritu Khanna MBBS MS FICOG
Director and Consultant
Department of Obstetrics and Gynecology
Khanna Medical Centre
Varanasi, Uttar Pradesh, India

S Sampathkumari MD
Professor and Head
Department of Obstetrics and Gynecology
Sri Muthukumaran Medical College Hospital and Research Institute
Chennai, Tamil Nadu, India

Sareena Gilvaz MD DGO
Professor and Head
Department of Obstetrics and Gynecology
Jubilee Mission Medical College
Thrissur, Kerala, India

Suchitra Pandit
MD DNB MRCOG FRCOG FICOG DFP BPharm MNAMS
Senior Consultant
Department of Obstetrics and Gynecology
Surya Group of Hospitals
Mumbai, Maharashtra, India

Sujata Dalvi MD DGO FCPS FICOG
Consultant
Department of Obstetrics and Gynecology
N Wadia/Gleneagles/Saifee/Bhatia Hospitals
Mumbai, Maharashtra, India

Sunita Tandulwadkar
MD (Obs and Gyne) FICS (Gyne-Endoscopy) FICOG
President, FOGSI (2025–2026)
Gynecological Endoscopist and ART & IVF Specialist
Head, Department of Obstetrics and Gynecology
Chief, IVF & Endoscopy Center
Ruby Hall Clinic, Pune
Founder and Medical Director
Solo Clinic IVF—A Center for Excellence in Infertility and Endoscopy, Pune
Founder and Medical Director
Solo Stem Cells—A Stem Cell Research and Application Center, Pune
Founder and Director
Alive Regenerative Wellness
Pune, Maharashtra, India

T Ramanidevi MD DGO FICS FICOG PhD
Director and Consultant
Department of Obstetrics and Gynecology
Ramakrishna Medical Centre LLP
Tiruchirappalli, Tamil Nadu, India

Uma Singh MBBS MS
Senior Technical Director, Maternal Health
Department of UP Technical Support Unit
University of Manitoba
Lucknow, Uttar Pradesh, India

Vidya Thobbi MD FICOG FKCOG
Professor
Department of Obstetrics and Gynecology
Al-Aameen Medical College
Rajiv Gandhi University of Health Sciences
Vijayapura, Karnataka, India

Vinita Kumari MBBS MD
Associate Professor
Department of Obstetrics and Gynecology
Nalanda Medical College and Hospital
Patna, Bihar, India

Preface

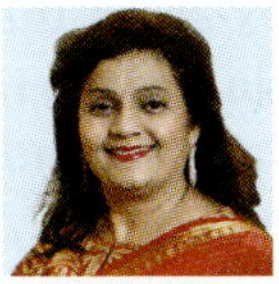

Editor-in-Chief
Sunita Tandulwadkar

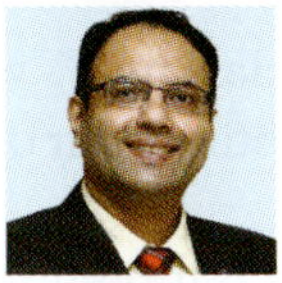

Editor
Ameya C Purandare

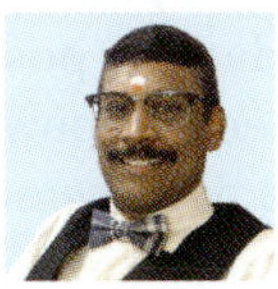

Editor
Palaniappan Narayanan

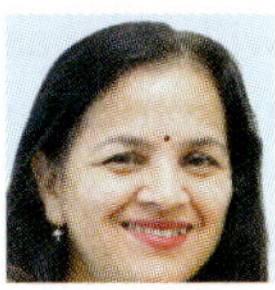

Expert
Suchitra Pandit

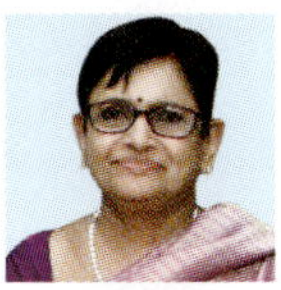

Expert
Jayam Kannan

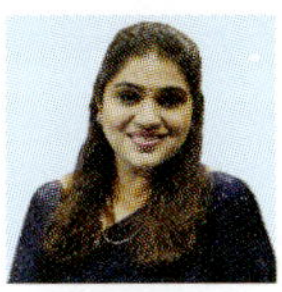

Convener
Pooja Lodha

In our pursuit of advancing women's health in India, establishing our own ethical evidence-based recommendations is essential. As the President of the Federation of Obstetric and Gynaecological Societies of India (FOGSI) 2025, I am delighted to present this *Ethical Evidence-Based Recommendations on Hypertensive Disorders of Pregnancy*, a comprehensive resource developed through the collaborative expertise of leading professionals across the country. While international organizations such as International Federation of Gynecology and Obstetrics (FIGO), American Society for Reproductive Medicine (ASRM), International Society of Human Reproduction (ISHRE), and Royal College of Obstetricians and Gynaecologists (RCOG) have established extensive recommendations, India has yet to provide a cohesive, evidence-backed framework tailored for hypertension in pregnancy. This publication bridges that gap, equipping Indian practitioners with practical, scientifically grounded recommendations for managing hypertension in pregnancy in diverse clinical settings.

This publication is organized to address all critical aspects of managing hypertension in pregnancy, beginning with "Definitions, Terminology, and Classifications", followed by a detailed exploration of "Epidemiology and Risk Factors" unique to Indian populations. We examine the "Etiology and Pathogenesis" to help clinicians understand the underlying mechanisms, and we include comprehensive insights on "Screening and Prediction of Preeclampsia" and "Preventive Strategies for Preeclampsia" for at-risk patients.

The resource continues with an in-depth look at "Clinical Features of Preeclampsia" and "Maternal Evaluation in Preeclampsia", guiding practitioners through the diagnostic and monitoring processes. In the section on "Therapeutics in Preeclampsia", we cover both "Antihypertensives" and "Anticonvulsants" to assist in selecting appropriate, evidence-based treatments.

"Decision to Deliver" and "Intrapartum Care in Preeclampsia" are addressed to support practitioners in managing complex cases through labor and delivery, with particular attention to "Preeclampsia and the Heart". This is followed by a focus on the "Complications of Preeclampsia and their Management", which include eclampsia, antepartum hemorrhage (APH), HELLP (hemolysis, elevated liver enzymes, low platelet count) syndrome, disseminated intravascular coagulation (DIC) with specific insights on its management, and pulmonary edema.

We also provide guidance on "Anesthesia in Preeclampsia", which addresses key considerations to ensure patient safety, promoting their overall health and well-being.

This publication represents FOGSI's commitment to equipping Indian gynecologists with the latest scientific advancements, framed within our cultural and clinical context. I am deeply grateful to the multidisciplinary team whose collaborative efforts have made these recommendations possible. We hope they become a trusted companion for practitioners, empowering them to deliver compassionate, evidence-based care in the management of hypertension in pregnancy.

Through this initiative, FOGSI reaffirms its dedication to advancing women's health and setting a new standard for ethical, informed care. We trust that these ethical evidence-based recommendations will serve as both a valuable guide and an inspiration for hypertension management across India.

Contents

1. **Definitions, Terminology, and Classifications 1**
   Ameya C Purandare, Parikshit Tank
2. **Epidemiology and Risk Factors.. 7**
   Neena Malhotra
3. **Etiology and Pathogenesis: Modern Understanding 14**
   Abha Rani Sinha, Vinita Kumari
4. **Screening and Prediction of Preeclampsia.................................. 21**
   K Aparna Sharma
5. **Preventive Strategies for Preeclampsia 32**
   Sujata Dalvi, Deepali Kapote
6. **Clinical Features of Preeclampsia 38**
   Munjal Pandya, Ashish Varma
7. **Maternal Evaluation in Preeclampsia... 42**
   Uma Singh
8. **Therapeutics in Preeclampsia 47**
   - 8.1 Hypertensive Disorders in Pregnancy 47
     Ritu Khanna
   - 8.2 Anticonvulsants 61
     Vidya Thobbi
9. **Decision to Deliver in Hypertensive Disorders in Pregnancy 73**
   Suchitra Pandit
10. **Intrapartum Care in Preeclampsia.. 80**
    Mitra Saxena
11. **Preeclampsia and the Heart.. 86**
    Palaniappan Narayanan
12. **Complications of Preeclampsia and their Management 96**
    - 12.1 Eclampsia 96
      S Sampathkumari
    - 12.2 Preeclampsia and APH 102
      Sareena Gilvaz
    - 12.3 HELLP Syndrome 103
      Komal N Chavan

12.4 **Disseminated Intravascular Coagulation** 113
T Ramanidevi

12.5 **Preeclampsia and Pulmonary Edema** 121
Prakash K Mehta

13. Anesthesia in Preeclampsia **136**
Hemant Mehta

CHAPTER 1

Definitions, Terminology, and Classifications

Ameya C Purandare, Parikshit Tank

Q1. What is preeclampsia?

Preeclampsia is a multisystem progressive disorder characterized by the new onset of hypertension and proteinuria or the new onset of hypertension plus significant end-organ dysfunction with or without proteinuria, typically presenting after 20 weeks of gestation or postpartum.

Diagnostic criteria for preeclampsia:
Systolic blood pressure >140 mm Hg and/or diastolic blood pressure >90 mm Hg on at least 2 occasions at least 4 hours apart after 20 weeks of gestation in a previously normotensive patient and the new onset of 1 or more of the following:*

- Proteinuria ≥0.3 g in a 24-hour urine specimen or protein/creatinine ratio ≥0.3 (30 mg/mmol) in a random urine specimen or dipstick ≥2+ if a quantitative measurement is unavailable
- Platelet count <100,000/μL
- Serum creatinine >1.1 mg/dL (97.2 μmol/L) or doubling *of* the creatinine concentration in the absence of other kidney disease
- Liver transaminases at least twice the upper limit of the normal concentrations for the local laboratory
- Pulmonary edema
- New-onset and persistent headache not accounted for by alternative diagnoses and not responding to usual doses of analgesics
- Visual symptoms (e.g., blurred vision, flashing lights or sparks, scotomata)

Preeclampsia is considered superimposed when it occurs in a patient with chronic hypertension. Superimposed preeclampsia is characterized by worsening or resistant hypertension (especially acutely), the new onset of proteinuria or a sudden increase in proteinuria, and/or significant new end-organ dysfunction in a patient with chronic hypertension. It typically occurs after 20 weeks of gestation or postpartum.

Definitions/diagnostic criteria for preeclampsia are generally similar worldwide except the International Society for the Study of Hypertension in Pregnancy (ISSHP) definition also includes signs of uteroplacental dysfunction (e.g., fetal growth restriction, abnormal angiogenic markers, abnormal umbilical artery Doppler, abruption, and fetal demise). The ISSHP also considers a platelet count <150,000/μL rather than <100,000/μL consistent with preeclampsia.

Note: *If systolic blood pressure is ≥160 mm Hg and/or diastolic blood pressure is ≥110 mm Hg, confirmation within minutes is sufficient.

Response to analgesia does not exclude the possibility of preeclampsia.

Contd...

Contd...

Source:
Adapted from:
1. American College of Obstetricians and Gynecologists (ACOG). ACOG Practice Bulletin No. 222: Gestational Hypertension and Preeclampsia. Obstet Gynecol. 2020;135:e237-60.
2. Magee LA, Brorwn MA, Hall DR, et al. The 2021 International Society for the Study of Hypertension in Pregnancy classification, diagnosis and management recommendations for international practice. Pregnancy Hypertens. 2022;27:148-69.

Q2. What is proteinuria?

Proteinuria is defines as a protein level of ≥0.3 g in a 24-hour urine specimen or protein/creatinine ratio ≥0.3 (30 mg/mmol) in a random urine specimen or dipstick ≥2+ if a quantitative measurement is unavailable.

Q3. What is classification of hypertensive disorders in pregnancy?

The International Society for the Study of Hypertension in Pregnancy (ISSHP) classification system for hypertensive disorders of pregnancy is as follows:

Prepregnancy or <20 weeks of gestation:
- *White-coat hypertension:* Systolic pressure ≥140 mm Hg and/or diastolic pressure ≥90 mm Hg when measured in the office or clinic, and blood pressure <135/85 mm Hg using home or ambulatory 24-hour blood pressure monitoring readings.
- *Masked hypertension:* Blood pressure <140/90 mm Hg at a clinic/office visit, but ≥135/85 mm Hg at other times outside the clinic/office.
- *Chronic hypertension:* Hypertension detected prepregnancy or before 20 weeks of gestation. Chronic hypertension may be essential hypertension (i.e., without a known secondary cause) or secondary hypertension (i.e., with a known secondary cause, e.g., kidney disease).

Pregnancy ≥20 weeks of gestation:
- *Gestational hypertension:* Hypertension de novo ≥20 weeks of gestation without proteinuria or other features suggestive of preeclampsia
- *Preeclampsia:* Gestational hypertension plus one or more of the following:
  - Proteinuria
  - Neurological complications (e.g., eclampsia, altered mental status, blindness, stroke, clonus, severe headaches, or persistent visual scotomata)
  - Pulmonary edema
  - Hematological complications (e.g., platelet count <150,000/μL, disseminated intravascular coagulation, hemolysis)
  - Acute kidney injury (such as creatinine ≥90 mmol/L or 1 mg/dL)

- Liver involvement (e.g., elevated transaminases such as ALT or AST >40 IU/L with or without right upper quadrant or epigastric abdominal pain)
- Uteroplacental dysfunction (e.g., placental abruption, angiogenic imbalance, fetal growth restriction, abnormal umbilical artery Doppler waveform analysis, or fetal death)

Q4. What is the clinical classification of preeclampsia?

The most commonly described clinical classification involves subtypes:

- Early onset (<34 weeks of gestation)
- Late onset (≥34 weeks of gestation)
- The clinical features overlap, but the spectrum of disease and outcomes differ: Early onset disease has been associated with more severe placental and maternal/fetal clinical findings and, in turn, poorer maternal/fetal outcomes.
- For this reason, it has been hypothesized that the two phenotypes have different origins and pathophysiologies.

Q5. What is gestational hypertension?

- *Gestational hypertension* refers to hypertension without proteinuria or other signs/symptoms of preeclampsia-related end-organ dysfunction that develops after 20 weeks of gestation in a patient with previously normal blood pressure.
- Up to 50% of these patients may ultimately develop signs and symptoms of preeclampsia.
- Development of proteinuria upgrades the diagnosis to preeclampsia.
- Even without proteinuria, patients who develop severe hypertension or other features of severe disease are managed in the same way as those with preeclampsia with severe features.
- True gestational hypertension should resolve by 12 weeks postpartum.

Q6. What is essential hypertension?

- Essential hypertension, also known as primary hypertension, is a type of high blood pressure that develops gradually over time and has no identifiable cause.
- It is the most common type of hypertension, affecting 85% of people with high blood pressure.

Q7. What is chronic hypertension?

- Hypertension detected prepregnancy or before 20 weeks of gestation. Chronic hypertension may be essential hypertension (i.e., without a known secondary cause) or secondary hypertension (i.e., with a known secondary cause, e.g., kidney disease).

- Preeclampsia superimposed upon chronic hypertension is diagnosed when preeclampsia occurs in a patient with preexisting chronic hypertension (hypertension that precedes pregnancy or is present on at least two occasions before the 20th week of gestation or persists longer than 12 weeks postpartum). It is characterized by worsening or resistant hypertension (especially acutely), the new onset of proteinuria or a sudden increase in proteinuria, and/or significant new end-organ dysfunction after 20 weeks of gestation or postpartum in a patient with chronic hypertension.

Q8. What is secondary hypertension?

- Secondary hypertension is a type of hypertension with an underlying and potentially reversible cause.
- It makes up only a small fraction (5–10%) of hypertensive cases.
- The prevalence of secondary hypertension varies by age and is more common in younger persons, with a prevalence close to 30% in those 18–40 years of age with hypertension.
- Extensive testing for secondary hypertension is not warranted in all patients with hypertension because of cost, low yield, and the potential for false-positive results; however, testing is recommended in patients younger than 30 years.

Q9. What is severe hypertension?

During pregnancy, hypertension is defined as systolic blood pressure ≥140 mm Hg and/or diastolic blood pressure ≥90 mm Hg. Severe hypertension is defined as systolic blood pressure ≥160 mm Hg and/or diastolic blood pressure ≥110 mm Hg.

Q10. What is severe preeclampsia?

Preeclampsia with severe features (formerly severe preeclampsia) is the subset of patients with preeclampsia who have severe hypertension and/or specific signs or symptoms of significant end-organ dysfunction that signify the severe end of the preeclampsia spectrum.

The specific criteria for diagnosis are listed in the Box here:

In a patient with preeclampsia, the presence of one or more of the following indicates a diagnosis of "preeclampsia with severe features":
Severe blood pressure elevation: Systolic blood pressure ≥160 mm Hg and/or diastolic blood pressure ≥110 mm Hg on 2 occasions at least 4 hours apart while the patient is on bed rest; however, antihypertensive therapy generally should be initiated upon confirmation of severe hypertension, in which case, criteria for severe blood pressure elevation can be satisfied without waiting until 4 hours have elapsed

Contd...

Contd...

Symptoms of central nervous system dysfunction: New-onset cerebral or visual disturbance, such as:

- Photopsia, scotomata, cortical blindness, retinal vasospasm
  and/or
- Severe headache (i.e., incapacitating, "the worst headache I've ever had") or headache that persists and progresses despite analgesic therapy with acetaminophen and not accounted for by alternative diagnoses

Hepatic abnormality:

- Impaired liver function not accounted for by another diagnosis and characterized by serum transaminase concentration >2 times the upper limit of the normal range
  and/or
- Severe persistent right upper quadrant or epigastric pain unresponsive to medication and not accounted for by an alternative diagnosis

Thrombocytopenia:

- Platelet count <100,000 platelets/μL

Kidney function impairment:

- Serum creatinine >1.1 mg/dL (97.2 μmol/L]
  and/or
- Doubling of the serum creatinine concentration in the absence of other kidney disease

Pulmonary edema

Source:

1. American College of Obstetricians and Gynecologists. ACOG Practice Bulletin No. 222: Gestational Hypertension and Preeclampsia. Obstet Gynecol. 2020;135(6):e237-60.

Q11. What is eclampsia?

- Eclampsia refers to the occurrence of new-onset, generalized, tonic–clonic seizures or coma in a patient with preeclampsia or gestational hypertension (in those cases where, in retrospect, a diagnosis of gestational hypertension was given before the patient went on to meet criteria for preeclampsia/eclampsia).
- Eclampsia is the convulsive manifestation of preeclampsia and one of several clinical manifestations at the severe end of the preeclampsia spectrum.
- Despite advances in detection and management, severe preeclampsia/eclampsia remains a common cause of maternal morbidity and death, especially in resource-limited areas.

Q12. What is HELLP syndrome?

- HELLP syndrome (*H*emolysis, *E*levated *L*iver enzymes, *L*ow *P*latelets) appears to be a subtype of preeclampsia with severe features in which hemolysis, elevated liver enzymes, and thrombocytopenia are the predominant features.

- Hypertension, central nervous system dysfunction, and/or renal dysfunction may also be present.
- The majority of patients, but not all, have hypertension (82–88%, although in some cases, the increase in blood pressure may be subtle initially) and/or proteinuria (86–100%).
- Rarely patients have neither; other diagnoses associated with similar laboratory abnormalities should be excluded before making the diagnosis of HELLP in these atypical patients.

Q13. What is mean arterial pressure?

Mean arterial pressure (MAP) is the average blood pressure during a cardiac cycle. It is a vital pressure that drives blood throughout the body's circulatory system.

Mean arterial pressure is usually calculated by adding one-third of the pulse pressure to the diastolic pressure:

- MAP = Diastolic BP + (Systolic – Diastolic BP)/3
  A normal MAP is around 90 mm Hg.

MAP is influenced by the cardiovascular and renal systems:

- *Cardiovascular system:* Determines MAP through cardiac output and systemic vascular resistance
- *Renal system:* Affects MAP through the renin–angiotensin–aldosterone system

Q14. What is PRES syndrome?

- Posterior reversible encephalopathy syndrome (PRES) is a rare clinic-radiological syndrome associated with acute changes in blood pressure during pregnancy.
- It is characterized symptomatically by headache, seizures, altered mental status, and visual blurring.
- Radiological changes are white matter vasogenic edema affecting the occipital and parietal lobes of the brain.
- It is being increasingly recognized due to increased institutional deliveries and advances in imaging particularly magnetic resonance imaging (MRI).

CHAPTER 2

Epidemiology and Risk Factors

Neena Malhotra

Q1. What is the prevalence of PE?

Draft recommendation: It is estimated that preeclampsia (PE) complicates 2–8% of pregnancies globally. The incidence of preeclampsia is influenced by race, ethnicity, and genetic predisposition. The prevalence varies globally, being higher in developed countries.

- *In the developed countries:* The prevalence of PE in developed countries is higher and varies between 1.0 and 5.6%. This is likely due to differences in classification, access to prenatal care and under-reporting in LMICs affecting prevalence data.
- *In the developing/LMIC:* The prevalence of PE is lower in developing and low-middle-income countries (LMIC) (except Sub-Saharan Africa) as compared to the high-income countries (HIC). The incidence of preeclampsia in hospital practice in India varies from 5 to 15%, and that of eclampsia is about 1.5%. In India, over the years, from 1976 to 2014, the risk of eclampsia ranged from 0.179 to 5%, with the average being 1.5%. A meta-analysis identified prevalence as 1 out of 11 pregnant women suffering from hypertensive disorders in India. The estimated overall pooled prevalence of hypertensive disorders of pregnancy (HDP) in India was found to be 11%. The higher prevalence in developing countries, including India, may be attributed to poverty, malnutrition, and poor access to health and obstetric care.

Summary of evidence: Global prevalence of preeclampsia has been reported at 4.6% of all deliveries between 2002 and 2010 with regional variation of 2–8% of all pregnancies. (Level III Evidence)

Evidence gaps: The exact prevalence of PE is not available from developing countries on account of under reporting.

Q2. What is the contribution of PE on maternal and perinatal outcomes?

Draft recommendations: Hypertensive disorders of pregnancy constitute one of the leading causes of maternal and perinatal mortality worldwide. PE is a major cause of maternal deaths second only to hemorrhage. PE accounts for 14% of maternal deaths (95% CI: 11.4–17.4). Maternal mortality is higher in a pre-eclamptic pregnancy than in a non-pre-eclamptic pregnancy [adjusted odds ratio (aOR) 3.73, 95% CI: 2.15–6.47]. The most common causes of maternal deaths include intracranial hemorrhage, HELLP syndrome, acute pulmonary edema, and acute renal failure.

Morbidity from PE is well recognized and may present later in life in the affected women. Patients with PE are at increased risk of future cardiovascular disease, metabolic syndrome, and chronic or end-stage renal disease. There is almost 20% risk of recurrence of hypertensive disorders of pregnancy (HDP), in women with chronic hypertension, besides 1.7–1.8-fold risk of major cardiovascular events and stroke in subsequent years. A recent meta-analysis demonstrated that women with previous PE have a RR of 3.13 (95% CI: 2.51–3.89) for future development of chronic hypertension, an OR of 2.28 (95% CI: 1.87–2.78) for future cardiovascular disease, and an OR of 1.8 (95% CI: 1.43–2.21) for cardiovascular accident. It has been observed that the earlier the onset of PE, the more severe the condition and the higher the risk of developing subsequent cardiovascular disease. Women with PE are also more likely to have microalbuminuria (a marker of renal damage) at 3–5 years after delivery. Data from prospective cohort study reported an association between PE and subsequent end-stage renal disease (RR: 4.7; 95% CI: 3.6–6.1).

- *Contribution to maternal mortality and morbidity in developed and developing countries:* Mortality from PE is variable globally, although maternal mortality is much lower in high-income countries than in developing countries, 16% of maternal deaths can be attributed to hypertensive disorders.

  In developed countries, PE accounts for approximately 16–26% of maternal deaths, as against 9% in developing world, although maternal mortality is much lower in high-income countries. In Latin America and the Caribbean, hypertensive disorders are responsible for almost 26% of maternal deaths, whereas in Africa and Asia, they contribute to 9% of deaths.
- *Contribution to perinatal mortality and morbidity in developed and developing countries:* The perinatal and neonatal complications are a consequence of placental hypoxia. The short-term complications include fetal growth restriction (FGR), oligohydramnios, intrauterine fetal death (IUFD), prematurity, low Apgar score, and need for intensive care at birth. Medically indicated preterm births are also the cause of neonatal deaths which are 2.7 times that of term birth.

  Infants born prematurely are at higher risk of neonatal mortality and morbidity, including necrotizing enterocolitis, retinopathy of prematurity, bronchopulmonary dysplasia, intraventricular hemorrhage, and neurodevelopmental impairment. The delayed complications include cerebral palsy, hearing and visual impairment, and low IQ. The

EPICure Study examined school age outcomes of all infants born at <26 weeks of gestation over a 5-year period in England. Cerebral palsy affected 6% of the survivors, whereas 41% had IQ tests more than two standard deviations (SDs) below the mean compared with schoolmates.

Summary of evidence: Overall hypertensive disorders of pregnancy (including preeclampsia) are the second most common cause (behind hemorrhage) of maternal deaths, accounting for 14% of maternal deaths (an estimated 62,000–77,000 deaths annually worldwide).

Perinatal mortality and morbidity are higher in PE pregnancy on account of prematurity, FGR requiring intensive neonatal care and long-term consequences including cerebral palsy, hearing and visual impairment besides lower IQ and learning disabilities.

Evidence gaps: The short- and long-term to perinatal morbidity of PE in developing countries including India is not exactly known as follow-up data from community on the newborn is not available.

Q3. What are the recognized risk factors for PE?

Draft recommendations: A variety of risk factors have been associated with increased probability of preeclampsia. Recognized risk factors include:

- *Previous history of preeclampsia:* It is the most predictive factor for the development of subsequent PE and is associated with an 8.4-fold increased risk compared with women with a previous uncomplicated pregnancy.
- *Maternal pre-existing comorbidities* including chronic hypertension [relative risk (RR) = 5.1], pregestational diabetes (RR = 3.7), antiphospholipid syndrome, and systemic lupus erythematosus (RR = 2.5) as per a recent systematic review. Women with both chronic hypertension and pregestational diabetes are eight times more likely to be diagnosed with PE.
- *Maternal age beyond 35 and age under 19 years:* Maternal age ≥35 years at delivery is associated with 1.2–3-fold increased risk of developing PE. Using multivariate logistic regression analysis, adjusting for confounders, the risk for late-onset PE increases by 4% with every 1-year increase in maternal age above 32 years.
- *Pregnancy after assisted reproductive techniques (ART)* doubles the risk of PE. In a cohort study, risk of PE was increased in women exposed to hyperestrogenic ovarian stimulation drugs as high levels of estrogens during implantation cause impaired placentation, reduced uteroplacental circulation, decreased number of uterine spiral arteries with vascular invasion. Pregnancy after ovum donation cycles is at incresed risk of PE.
- *Multifetal gestations:* PE is 2.9 times more likely to develop in a multifetal pregnancy.

- *Low maternal birth weight:* Women with low birth weight (<2,500 g) have double the risk of developing PE (OR: 2.3, 95% CI: 1.0–5.3) when compared with women who weighed 2,500–2,999 g at birth.
- *High pre-pregnancy BMI, especially beyond ≥30 kg/m^2*, increases the risk of developing PE by 2–4-fold.
- *Maternal kidney disease:* PE may occur frequently in pregnant women with chronic kidney disease, lupus nephropathy, and diabetic nephropathy. For women with diabetes, proteinuria of either 190–499 mg/day or +2 on urine dipstick at booking is associated with a significantly higher risk.
- *Family history of PE:* Daughters or sisters of women with PE are 3–4 times more likely to develop the condition than women without a family history.
- *Short duration of sperm exposure:* Conception within the first 4 months of a couple's sexual relationship carries a high risk (incidence of 40–50%) that hypertension will complicate the pregnancy. However, this risk significantly decreased in women after at least 1 year of cohabitation before conception.
- *Interpregnancy interval:* Both short and long interpregnancy intervals are associated with an increased risk. Interpregnancy intervals <12 months or >72 months are associated with higher risk of PE development compared with interpregnancy intervals of 12–23 months.
- *Mental disorders:* Depression and anxiety in the first trimester of pregnancy are known to increase the risk of preeclampsia by twofold to threefold.

Summary of evidence: Despite recognized risk factors, PE may develop in women without identifiable risk factors.

Evidence gaps: Risk factors are identified from women in HIC. Risk profile of women from Low- and Middle Income Countries (LMIC) is not available in particular factors such as anemia, malaria, and prior health during adolescence.

Q4. What are the emerging risk factors for PE?

Draft recommendations:

Emerging factors for PE include:

- Residence at high altitudes (>2,700 m) is at increased risk of preeclampsia (for example, Colorado, USA, 33% of pregnancies; Peru, 22% of pregnancies; Bolivia, 20% of pregnancies; as against worldwide prevalence, 4.6%). Maternal hypoxia consequent to high altitude affects multiple physiological systems, including placenta/decidual vasculature, resulting in increased rate of preeclampsia.
- Air pollution with poor air quality is emerging risk factor for PE. Associations between exposure to ambient particulate matter and nitrogen dioxide and increased PE have been reported.

- Genetic involvement has been recognized with mother, daughters, and sisters reporting a threefold to fourfold higher risk. Women lacking the activating KIR (killer-cell immunoglobulin-like receptor; AA genotype) are at greater risk of preeclampsia when the fetus expresses the HLA-C2 genotype. A genome-wide association meta-analysis of European and Central Asian mothers and offspring identified three sequence variants associated with PE: one in FLT1 gene of individuals born of PE pregnancies and two in the FTO (encoding α-ketoglutarate-dependent dioxygenase) and ZNF831 (encoding zinc finger protein 831) genes in women with preeclamptic pregnancies. The soluble form of FLT1 (sFLT1) is a placental-released anti-angiogenic factor used in diagnostic tests for PE. Variants in FTO and ZNF831 are associated with blood pressure, obesity, BMI, and type 2 diabetes.

Summary of evidence: Newer factors are evolving as risk for developing PE. Factors including high altitude and air pollutions are emerging risk factors for PE, besides role of newer genetic markers including some HLA and KIR genotype.

Evidence gaps: Emerging genetic factors, including FLT1, FTO, and ZNF831, need to be validated in larger studies and across communities over the globe.

Q5. What is the gestosis scoring for PE?

Draft recommendations: This scoring is based on existing and emerging risk factors that incorporates past history and index pregnancy factors, obstetrical and medical to identify women at risk of PE. It is an effective and feasible prediction policy and easy to use. The process of risk scoring includes factors given in **Table 1**.

TABLE 1: Gestosis scoring for PE [FOGSI-GESTOSIS-ICOG Hypertensive Disorders in Pregnancy (HDP) 2019 guidelines, for Indian population].

Risk factor	*Score*
Woman born as small for gestational age	1
Maternal anemia	1
Age older than 35 years	1
Age younger than 19 years	1
Obesity (BMI >30)	1
Nulligravida	1
Short duration of paternity (cohabitation)	1
Family history of preeclampsia	1
Family history of cardiovascular disease	1

Contd...

Contd...

Risk factor	*Score*
Polycystic ovary syndrome	1
Inter-pregnancy interval more than 5 years	1
Assisted reproductive (IVF/ICSI) treatment	1
Maternal hypothyroidism	1
Chronic vascular disease	1
Excessive weight gain during pregnancy	1
MAP >85	1
Gestational diabetes mellitus	2
Obesity (BMI >40)	2
Multiple pregnancy	2
Hypertensive disease during previous pregnancy	2
Pregestational diabetes mellitus	3
Chronic hypertension	3
Mental disorder (e.g., schizophrenia)	3
Inherited/acquired thrombophilia	3
Maternal chronic kidney disease	3
Autoimmune disease (SLE/APLAS/RA)	3
Assisted reproductive (OD) treatment	3

When total score is ≥3; a pregnant woman should be marked as "At risk for PE".

Summary of evidence: Gestosis scoring is easy, feasible, and can be done by any healthcare worker to identify women at risk of PE.

Evidence gaps: Needs to be validated through large community-based data and scored in light of ACOG, NICE guidelines.

BIBLIOGRAPHY

1. Abalos E, Cuesta C, Grosso AL, et al. Global and regional estimates of preeclampsia and eclampsia: a systematic review. Eur J Obstet Gynecol Reprod Biol. 2013;170:1-7.
2. Bartsch E, Medcalf KE, Park AL, et al. Clinical risk factors for pre-eclampsia determined in early pregnancy: systematic review and meta-analysis of large cohort studies. BMJ. 2016;353:i1753.
3. Brown MC, Best KE, Pearce MS, et al. Cardiovascular disease risk in women with pre-eclampsia: Systematic review and meta-analysis. Eur J Epidemiol. 2013;28:1-19.

4. Dhinwa M, Gawande K, Jha N, et al. Prevalence of Hypertensive disorders in pregnancy in India. A Systematic Review and Meta-analysis. J Med Evidence. 2021;2(2):105-12.
5. Khan KS, Wojdyla D, Say L, et al. WHO analysis of causes of maternal death: a systematic review. Lancet. 2006;367:1066-74.
6. Marlow N, Wolke D, Bracewell MA, et al. Neurologic and developmental disability at six years of age after extremely preterm birth. N Engl J Med. 2005;352:9-19.
7. Moore LG. Hypoxia and reproductive health: reproductive challenges at high altitude: fertility, pregnancy and neonatal well-being. Reproduction. 2021;161(1):F81-F90.
8. Steegers EA, von Dadelszen P, Duvekot JJ, et al. Pre-eclampsia. Lancet. 2010;376:631-44.
9. Steinthorsdottir V, McGinnis R, Williams NO, et al. Genetic predisposition to hypertension is associated with preeclampsia in European and Central Asian women. Nat Commun. 2020;11:5976.
10. Vikse BE, Irgens LM, Leivestad T, et al. Preeclampsia and the risk of end-stage renal disease. N Engl J Med. 2008;359:800-9.

3

CHAPTER

Etiology and Pathogenesis: Modern Understanding

Abha Rani Sinha, Vinita Kumari

Q1. Describe current concepts in etiology of preeclampsia.

Multiple etiological factors may be associated with preeclampsia. These include uteroplacental ischemia, maternal infection and inflammation, maternal intestinal dysbiosis, maternal obesity, and endocrine disorders.

Uteroplacental ischemia: In normal pregnancies, invading trophoblastic cells migrate through the decidua and part of the myometrium to reach both the endothelium and highly muscular tunica media of the spiral arteries. As a result, these vessels undergo transformation from small muscular arterioles to high-capacitance low-resistance vessels, which facilitate increased blood flow to the placenta compared with other areas of the uterus.

In preeclampsia, invading trophoblast fails to penetrate the myometrial segment, the spiral arteries fail to develop into large, tortuous vascular channels, the vessels remain narrow, resulting in placental hypoperfusion and relatively hypoxic trophoblast tissue. This abnormal placentation has been associated with development of preeclampsia and multiple other adverse pregnancy outcomes.

A systematic review and meta-analysis showed that placental lesions contributed to maternal vascular malperfusion. Placental infarction, failure of physiologic transformation of the spiral arteries, and acute atherosis were found to be fourfold to sevenfold higher in women with preeclampsia than in those with a normal pregnancy.

Maternal infection and inflammation:

Urinary tract infection: Microbial colonization of the maternal urinary tract has been found to be associated with preeclampsia. A systematic review observed that urinary tract infections are closely associated with preeclampsia.

SARS CoV-2 infection: SARS-CoV-2 infection can be causally linked to preeclampsia. The mechanism proposed is endothelial dysfunction.

A recent meta-analysis demonstrated that SARS-CoV-2 infection during pregnancy is associated with a significant increase in the odds of developing preeclampsia, preeclampsia with severe features, eclampsia, and HELLP syndrome.

Maternal intestinal dysbiosis: Human gut microbiota changes have been reported in preeclampsia, which may persist 6 weeks postpartum.

The changes include a reduction in microbial burden with *Firmicutes, Clostridia, Clostridiales,* and *Ruminococcus* and an increase in *Bacteroidetes, Proteobacteria, Actinobacteria, Bacteroidia, Gamma-proteobacteria,* and Enterobacteriaceae.

Gestational diabetes mellitus, metabolic syndrome, and obesity: Gestational diabetes mellitus (GDM) is found to be an independent risk factor for preeclampsia. A retrospective cohort study of 212,463 women showed that the presence of prepregnancy metabolic syndrome was associated with an increased risk of preeclampsia. A meta-analysis of 29 prospective cohort studies comprising 1,980,761 participants and 67,075 cases of preeclampsia showed that maternal obesity was significantly associated with the development of preeclampsia.

Cushing's syndrome: Cushing's syndrome is associated with an increased risk of preeclampsia.

Adenomyosis: Women with adenomyosis are at significantly increased risk of developing preeclampsia. The contributing factors are poor placentation and endothelial inflammation.

Q2. What is new in pathogenesis?

Preeclampsia is an enigmatic disorder in which multiple and sometimes overlapping pathologic processes activate a common pathway comprising of endothelial cell activation, intravascular inflammation, and syncytiotrophoblast stress.

Defects in trophoblast differentiation: Trophoblast differentiation involves alteration in expression of cytokines, adhesion molecules, extracellular matrix molecules, metalloproteinases, and the class Ib major histocompatibility complex molecule, human leukocyte antigen (HLA-G).

During normal differentiation, invading trophoblasts alter their adhesion molecule expression from those that are characteristic of epithelial cells integrin alpha-6/beta-1, alpha-V/beta-5, and E-cadherin to those of endothelial cells integrin alpha-1/beta-1, alpha-V/beta-3, and VE-cadherin, a process referred to as pseudovasculogenesis. Trophoblasts obtained from patients with preeclampsia do not show upregulated adhesion molecule expression or pseudovasculogenesis.

The decidual cells of patients who go on to develop preeclampsia have greater soluble fms-like tyrosine kinase-1 (sFlt-1) expression during decidualization, which may contribute to failed spiral artery modification and shallow placentation. Decidual natural killer (NK) cells contribute to spiral artery remodeling and NK dysfunction has been implicated in the genesis of preeclampsia.

Defective placental perfusion: Hypoperfusion in preeclampsia primarily results from defective spiral artery remodeling.

Hypoperfusion becomes more pronounced as pregnancy progresses since the abnormal uterine vasculature is unable to accommodate the normal increase in blood flow and increased metabolic demand of the fetus and placenta. Vascular lesions that may develop as pregnancy advances include atherosis fibrinoid necrosis, thrombosis, sclerotic narrowing of arterioles, and placental infarction.

Hypoperfusion/ischemia results in release of antiangiogenic factors, such as sFlt-1 and soluble endoglin (sEng) that bind or inhibit proangiogenic factors VEGF, placental growth factor (PlGF). This results in widespread maternal vascular inflammation, vascular injury, and endothelial dysfunction, leading to hypertension, vasospasm, platelet adhesion and aggregation, proteinuria, and the other clinical manifestations of preeclampsia.

Obesity: Preeclampsia is associated with elevated circulating interleukin (IL)-6 and adipose-derived leptin levels as well as threefold and fivefold increases in IL-6 and leptin receptor expression, respectively, in Hofbauer cells from preeclamptic placentas.

In vitro fertilization (IVF): Compared with spontaneous conception, pregnancies after IVF have been associated with a higher risk of adverse pregnancy outcomes, including preeclampsia and fetal growth restriction. The strength of association is greatest in oocyte donation pregnancies.

Role of angiogenic and antiangiogenic factors: sFlt-1, VEGF, and PlGF

A variety of proangiogenic [vascular endothelial growth factor (VEGF), placental growth factor (PlGF)] and antiangiogenic factors [soluble fms-like tyrosine kinase-1 (sFlt-1)] are released by the developing placenta, and the balance among these factors is important for normal placental development. Increased placental production of antiangiogenic factors disturbs this balance and results in the systemic endothelial dysfunction characteristic of preeclampsia. Compared with normotensive controls, circulating levels of sFlt-1 levels are increased and free VEGF and free PlGF are decreased in patients with preeclampsia.

Studies using banked sera showed that these patients had decreases in PlGF and VEGF levels well before the onset of clinical disease. Multiple studies have shown that alterations in both sFlt-1 and PlGF correlate with adverse maternal and neonatal outcomes associated with preeclampsia. In patients with preeclampsia at term (i.e., ≥37 weeks), an abnormal angiogenic profile (sFlt-1:PlGF) also identifies those with excess inflammatory profiles and at higher risk of adverse outcomes.

Decreased production of endothelial-derived vasodilators, such as nitric oxide and prostacyclin, and increased production of vasoconstrictors, such as endothelins and thromboxanes, may also play a role in the vascular changes in preeclampsia.

Impaired flow-mediated vasodilation and impaired acetylcholine mediated vasorelaxation may contribute to the vasoconstriction in patients with preeclampsia.

Genetic factors: Most cases of preeclampsia are sporadic, but genetic factors are thought to play a role in disease susceptibility.

Genomic data:

PAI-1 4G/5G polymorphism: A meta-analysis of studies of PAI-1 4G/5G polymorphism (recessive model) showed strong consistent evidence for an association with risk for preeclampsia.

A large genome-wide association study (GWAS) of offspring from preeclamptic pregnancies identified a genome-wide susceptibility locus near the *Flt1* gene encoding Fms-like tyrosine kinase 1 and provided convincing replication in an independent cohort. These findings were confirmed in additional European cohorts. This GWAS finding provides compelling evidence that alterations in chromosome 13 near the *Flt1* locus in the human fetal genome are causal in the development of preeclampsia.

Q3. Describe pathophysiology of neurological changes in preeclampsia.

Neurological complications are the forerunners of all the complications leading to mortality due to preeclampsia, accounting for 30–70% of all deaths due to preeclampsia. The pathophysiological neurological changes seen in maternal brain are impaired cerebral autoregulation in chronic hypertension and preeclamptic cases both in animal and human clinical studies but not in normotensive.

By cerebral autoregulation, cerebral arterioles change accordingly and ensure a constant flow of blood to the brain and hyperperfusion injury is prevented, but in preeclampsia, this autoregulation is lost.

Permeability of blood–brain barrier is increased leading to cerebral edema mostly seen in eclampsia but sometimes also in preeclampsia. This is due to increased neuroinflammatory factors especially TNF-α.

Moreover, preeclampsia is associated with microvascular disease leading to long-term cognitive effects and risk of stroke.

Q4. What are the renal changes in pre-eclampsia?

Preeclampsia and preeclampsia-associated renal dysfunction (PARD) are associated with morbidities during pregnancy resulting in potentially devastating maternal and fetal outcomes. In preeclampsia, kidney is affected both functionally and morphologically. It may cause renal function derangement due to acute kidney injury, endothelial damage, and podocyte loss. There is decrease in renal hemodynamics and increase in urinary protein excretion. These changes are due to glomerular lesions. The glomerular lesions are characteristic of preeclampsia and can be clearly differentiated from hypertensive and other nephropathies.

As the disease progresses, placental hypoxia leads to release of stress mediators resulting in endothelial cell damage of the glomerulus.

As the disease progresses, the GFR decreases when compared to normal pregnancy. The antiangiogenic mediators released cause endothelial injury, and thereby glomerular injury due to inflammation, vasoconstriction, and disruption in integrity of the glomerulus.

This occurs because placental soluble fms-like tyrosine kinase-1 (sFLT-1) and soluble endoglin (sEng) produced due to placental hypoxia antagonize the effects of podocyte vascular endothelial growth factor (VEGF) on the renal ECs. Also, increased production of reactive oxygen species (ROS) due to the oxidative stress associated with placental ischemia leads to further damage, the glomerular endothelial cells become swollen along with fenestrae and capillary lumen occlusion. There is hypertrophy of the intracapillary cells, hypertrophy of the cytoplasmic organelles in endothelial cells, mesangial cells, and especially the lysosomes. This is called the glomerular endotheliosis. It mostly occurs due to the thrombotic microangiopathy.

Q5. What are the hepatic changes in pre-eclampsia?

Hepatic biopsy in preeclampsia shows ischemia, periportal hemorrhage, deposits of microvesicular fat, and fibrinogen deposition. These findings indicate endothelial cell injury and exposure to subendothelial collagen. There is evidence of increased fibrosis also.

The endothelial cell injury causes decreased prostacyclin and increased thromboxane. The resultant vasoconstriction of hepatic vessels leads to hypoxia of hepatocytes. Hypoxia in turn leads to degeneration and necrosis of hepatocytes.

As a result of hypoxia, necrosis and degeneration liver enzymes are raised in preeclampsia. Aspartate aminotransferase is more likely to be increased as compared to alanine transaminase. In more severe forms of disease, HELLP syndrome may occur. Lactate dehydrogenase may be elevated due to hepatic damage and hemolysis may also occur, which in turn leads to raised bilirubin. Coagulopathy may occur in severe liver damage.

Summary: The understanding of pathogenesis has increased dramatically in the past 30 years. It is no longer considered merely a hypertensive disorder with renal involvement, rather abundant evidence now supports preeclampsia as a pregnancy specific multisystemic syndrome. Overlapping pathologic processes activate a common pathway comprising endothelial cell activation, intravascular inflammation, and syncytiotrophoblast stress.

Research gaps: The pathophysiology of preeclampsia suddenly appearing at near term is not explained by abnormal placentation and needs further research.

BIBLIOGRAPHY

1. Alese MO, Moodley J, Naicker T. Preeclampsia and HELLP syndrome, the role of liver. J Matern Fetal Neonatal Med. 2021;34:117-23.
2. American College of Obstetricians and Gynecologists. Gestational Hypertension and Preeclampsia: ACOG Practice Bulletin: Number 222. Obstet Gynecol. 2020;135:e237-60.
3. Beckers KF, Sones JL. Maternal microbiome and the hypertensive disorder of pregnancy, preeclampsia. Am J Physiol Heart Circ Physiol. 2020;318:H1-h10.
4. Caimari F, Valassi E, Garbayo P, et al. Cushing's syndrome and pregnancy outcomes: a systematic review of published cases. Endocrine. 2017;55:555-63.
5. Chaiworapongsa T, Romero R, Gomez-Lopez N, Suksai M, Gallo DM, Jung E, et al. Preeclampsia at term: evidence of disease heterogeneity based on the profile of circulating cytokines and angiogenic factors. Am J Obstet Gynecol. 2024;230:450.e1-450.e18.
6. Chih HJ, Elias FTS, Gaudet L, et al. Assisted reproductive technology and hypertensive disorders of pregnancy: systematic review and meta-analyses. BMC Pregnancy Childbirth. 2021;21:449.
7. Conde-Agudelo A, Romero R. SARS-COV-2 infection during pregnancy and risk of preeclampsia: a systematic review and meta-analysis. Am J Obstet Gynecol. 2022;226(1):68-89.e3.
8. Elharram M, Dayan N, Kaur A, Landry T, Pilote L. Long term cognitive impairment after preeclampsia: A systematic review and meta-analysis. Obstet Gynecol. 2018;132:355-64.
9. Falco ML, Sivanathan J, Laoreti A, Thilaganathan B, Khalil A. Placental histopathology associated with pre-eclampsia: systematic review and meta-analysis. Ultrasound Obstet Gynecol. 2017;50:295-301.
10. Giannakou K, Evangelou E, Papatheodorou SI. Genetic and non-genetic risk factors for pre-eclampsia: umbrella review of systematic reviews and meta-analyses of observational studies. Ultrasound Obstet Gynecol. 2018;51:720.
11. Guilbaud L, Santulli P, Studer E, et al. Impact of oocyte donation on perinatal outcome in twin pregnancies. Fertil Steril. 2017;107:948.
12. Horton J, Sterrenburg M, Lane S, et al. Obstetric and perinatal outcomes of women with adenomyosis and endometriosis: a systematic review and meta-analysis. Hum Reprod Update. 2019;25:592-63.
13. Johnson KM, Hacker MR, Thornton K, et al. Association between in vitro fertilization and ischemic placental disease by gestational age. Fertil Steril. 2020;114:579.
14. Kikas T, Inno R, Ratnik K, et al. C-allele of rs4769613 Near FLT1 Represents a High-Confidence Placental Risk Factor for Preeclampsia. Hypertension. 2020;76:884-91.
15. Levine RJ, Maynard SE, Qian C, et al. Circulating angiogenic factors and the risk of preeclampsia. N Engl J Med. 2004;350:672-83.
16. Maeda KJ, McClung DM, Showmaker KC, et al. Endothelial cell disruption drives increased blood brain permeability and cerebral edema in the DahlSS/jr rat model of superimposed preeclampsia. Am J Physiol Heart Circ Physiol. 2021;320(2):H535-48.

17. McGinnis R, Steinthorsdottir V, Williams NO, et al. Variants in the fetal genome near FLT1 are associated with risk of preeclampsia. Nat Genet. 2017;49:1255-60.
18. Moreno-Sepulveda J, Checa MA. Correction to: Risk of adverse perinatal outcomes after oocyte donation: a systematic review and meta-analysis. J Assist Reprod Genet. 2020; 37:239.
19. Ozmen A, Nwabuobi C, Tang Z, et al. Leptin-Mediated Induction of IL-6 Expression in Hofbauer Cells Contributes to Preeclampsia Pathogenesis. Int J Mol Sci. 2023;25:135.
20. Sahu MB, Deepak V, Gonzales SK, et al. Decidual cells from women with preeclampsia exhibit inadequate decidualization and reduced sFlt1 suppression. Pregnancy Hypertens. 2019;15:64-71.
21. Sani HM, Vahed SZ, Ardalan M. Preeclampsia: A close look at renal dysfunction. Biomed Pharmacother. 2019;109:408-16.
22. Spradley FT. Metabolic abnormalities and obesity's impact on the risk for developing preeclampsia. Am J Physiol Regul Integr Comp Physiol. 2017;312:R5-r12.
23. Wang Z, Wang P, Liu H, et al. Maternal adiposity as an independent risk factor for pre-eclampsia: a meta-analysis of prospective cohort studies. Obes Rev. 2013;14:508-21.
24. Yan L, Jin Y, Hang H, et al. The association between urinary tract infection during pregnancy and preeclampsia: a meta-analysis. Medicine (Baltimore). 2018;97:e12192.

CHAPTER 4

Screening and Prediction of Preeclampsia

K Aparna Sharma

KEY QUESTIONS

1. Should universal screening for PE be offered to all pregnant women in the first trimester?
2. What is the efficacy of history-based screening?
3. What is the added role of blood pressure to history-based screening?
4. What is the added role of uterine artery Doppler to maternal factors?
5. What is the added role of biochemistry to maternal factors and biophysical factors?
6. What is the ideal protocol for PE screening?
7. What is the pragmatic protocol for PE screening?
8. What is the role of biochemical markers for prediction of preeclampsia in the second and third trimester?

INTRODUCTION

Preeclampsia (PE) is a multisystem disorder which is characterized by new onset of hypertension along with significant proteinuria after 20 weeks' gestation. This disorder affects 2–8% of pregnant women and is one of the leading causes of maternal and perinatal morbidity and mortality. Preeclampsia can cause many maternal adverse effects, including impairment of hepatorenal and coagulation systems and in severe form, it can cause pulmonary edema, eclampsia, brain hemorrhage, etc. In fetal complications, fetal growth restriction, preterm birth, or stillbirth is seen because of uteroplacental insufficiency. Moreover, preeclampsia is associated with an increased risk of long-term cardiovascular and chronic diseases in both the mothers and their children from the affected pregnancy. Women with preeclampsia are also at elevated risk for chronic hypertension, future cardiovascular disease, stroke, metabolic syndromes, cognitive impairment, and chronic end-stage renal disease later in life. It has been proposed to further sub-classify preeclampsia according to gestational age at delivery because evidence suggests that early- and late-onset disease have different pathophysiologic and etiologic pathways. Early-onset preeclampsia is associated with a higher risk of adverse maternal and perinatal outcomes.

Q1. Should universal screening for PE be offered to all pregnant women in the first trimester?

Draft Recommendation 1.1: All pregnant women should be offered preeclampsia screening in early pregnancy (between 11 and 14 weeks)

Need for screening and prediction: PE can be subdivided into early-onset PE with delivery <34 weeks' gestation and late-onset PE with delivery more than 34 weeks. It is the early-onset PE which is of great concern because it is associated with great amount of neonatal morbidity in terms of prematurity. It becomes imperative to identify early pregnancies at high risk of early-onset PE and to undertake necessary measures to decrease the effect of defective placentation and reduce the prevalence of the disease and, therefore, shift in pyramid of antenatal care to first trimester is required. The need for screening for preeclampsia is important because there exists an evidence-based strategy to prevent it. Low-dose aspirin for prophylactic use for prevention of preeclampsia has been investigated by a number of researchers. If the treatment is started at an early gestation, there is a significant reduction in early-onset PE and this is supported by various study groups and various international agencies. Also, identification of an "at risk" group will allow tailored antenatal surveillance to anticipate and recognize the onset of the clinical syndrome and manage it promptly.

Q2. What is the efficacy of history-based screening?

Draft Recommendation 2.1: *Although the history-based screening has a low detection rate, it is recommended to include this as a part of routine prenatal care.*

Screening by maternal history: Most of the professional bodies recommend that at the booking visit detailed history should be taken and have issued guidelines for same **(Table 1)**. Estimated DR of PE requiring delivery before 34, 37, and 42 week's gestation in screening by maternal factors are about 51, 43, and 40% respectively at FPR of 10%. In spite of such low detection rates, most of the professional bodies including American College of Obstetricians and Gynecologists recommend taking a detailed medical history only to assess a patient's risks for developing preeclampsia **(Table 1)**.

TABLE 1: Risk factors to be considered while taking history in first trimester.

ACOG 2018	
High risk	***Moderate risk***
• Previous pregnancy with PE • Chronic hypertension • Systemic lupus erythematosus • Type 1 or type 2 diabetes mellitus • Renal disease • Multifetal gestation • Antiphospholipid syndrome	• Nulliparity • Age >35 year • Interpregnancy interval >10 year • BMI >30 kg/m^2 • Family history of PE (mother or sister) • History of SGA or adverse outcome • Sociodemographic characteristics (African American race or low socioeconomic status)

Q3. What is the added role of blood pressure to history-based screening?

Draft Recommendation 3.1: *Calculation of mean arterial pressure in the first trimester and combining with maternal factors improves the detection significantly for preterm preeclampsia.*

Blood pressure: Women who subsequently develop PE have higher systolic blood pressure and MAP before the onset of clinical disease. MAP is calculated by adding one-third of pulse pressure to the diastolic pressure. The correct method of measurement is that MAP should be measured by validated automated devices with women in sitting position with back supported and legs uncrossed. Arms should be well supported at the level of their heart, and an appropriate-sized adult cuff (small <22 cm, normal 22–32 cm, or large 33–42 cm) should be used. After rest for 5 minutes, BP is measured in both arms simultaneously. Two sets of recordings are made at 1-minute intervals. The four sets of SBP and DBP measurements are needed for input into the risk calculator. If MAP is taken in first trimester along with maternal characteristics, the detection rate of preeclampsia goes up to 74% for early preeclampsia and 49% for late preeclampsia with a false positive rate of 10%. If we measure MAP in both first and second trimester, we have a detection rate of 84% for early preeclampsia, and 53% for late preeclampsia with a false positive rate of 10%.

Q4. What is the added role of uterine artery Doppler to maternal factors?

Draft Recommendation 4.1: *Addition of uterine artery Doppler pulsatility index between 11 and 13 weeks improves the detection rate achieved for preeclampsia over and above the maternal factors and mean arterial pressure.*

Uterine artery Doppler: The spiral arteries undergo a transformation to low-resistance vessels by trophoblastic invasion and increases blood flow in the placental bed in pregnancy. If this mechanism fails, it leads to defective placentation. The uterine artery PI MoM is significantly increased at 11–13 weeks' gestation in women who subsequently develop PE. The addition of uterine artery PI to maternal factors improves the DR from 51 to 75% and 43 to 55% at FPR of 10% for PE requiring delivery before 34 and 37 weeks' gestation. A sagittal section of the uterus should be obtained by using trans-abdominal ultrasonography and the cervical canal and internal cervical os needs to be identified. Color flow mapping is used to identify each uterine artery along the side of the cervix and uterus at the level of the internal os. Pulsed wave Doppler is then used with the sampling gate set at 2 mm to cover the whole vessel and care should be taken to ensure that the angle of insolation is less than 30. When three similar consecutive waveforms are obtained, the PI is measured and the mean PI of the left and right arteries is calculated. It is important to ensure that the peak systolic velocity is greater than 60 cm/s **(Fig. 1)**.

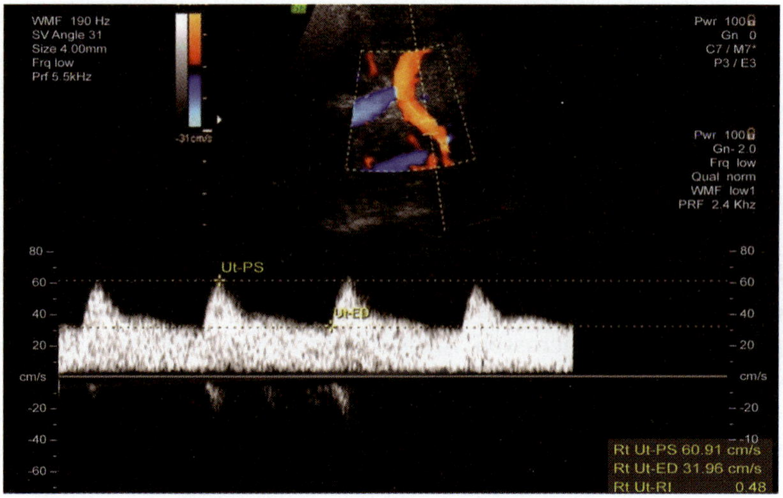

Fig. 1: Measurement of uterine artery PI.

Q5. What is the added role of biochemistry to maternal factors and biophysical factors?

Draft Recommendation 5.1: *Addition of placental growth factor to maternal factors and biophysical parameters between 11 and 13 weeks can significantly improve the detection rates for preterm preeclampsia.*

Draft Recommendation 5.2: *Addition of PAPP-A to maternal factors and mean arterial pressure can significantly improve the detection rate in those cases where uterine artery Doppler has not been performed.*

A plethora of biochemical markers have been investigated for the prediction of PE which includes PlGF, PAPP A, inhibin-A and activin-A, PP13, disintegrin and metalloprotease 12 (ADAM12), cystatin C, pentraxin 3, P-selectin, fetal hemoglobin. Maternal serum PAPP-A and PlGF are two biochemical markers that are useful markers not only for aneuploidy screening but also for predicting preeclampsia. Pregnancy-associated plasma protein-A is a syncytiotrophoblast-derived metalloproteinase, which enhances the mitogenic function of the insulin-like growth factors by cleaving the complex formed between such growth factors and their binding proteins. PAPP-A plays an important role in placental growth and development, therefore, low serum PAPP-A is associated with a higher incidence of PE. Placental growth factor (PlGF) is a glycosylated dimeric glycoprotein, which is a member of the vascular endothelial growth factor subfamily. PlGF is pro-angiogenic and has been speculated to play a role in normal pregnancy, and decrease in its level has been implicated in development of PE **(Fig. 2)**. These reduced levels of serum PlGF are evident from both the first- and second-trimesters of pregnancy. Both PAPP-A and PlGF have shown to be affected

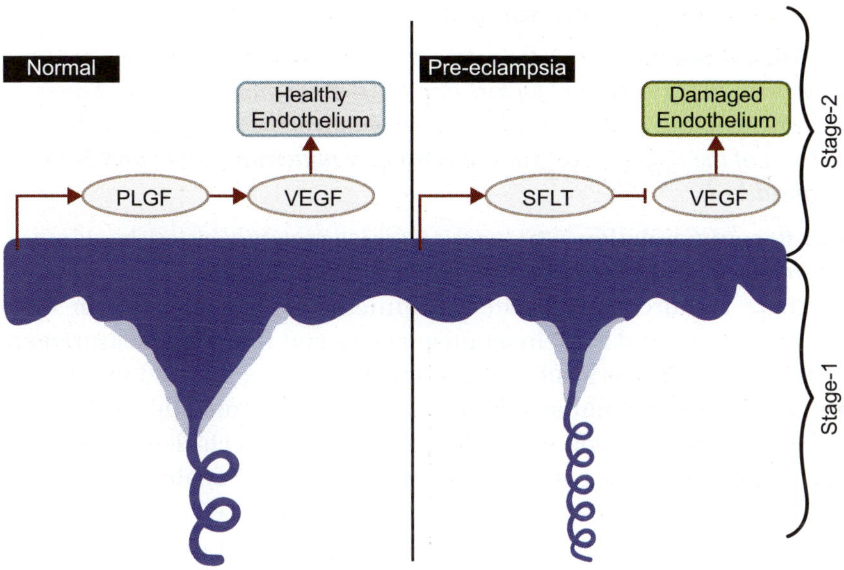

Fig. 2: Pathogenesis of preeclampsia (stagewise).

by gestational age at screening, maternal weight, racial origin, cigarette smoking, conception by IVF, nulliparity, and pre-existing diabetes mellitus. In addition, serum PlGF is also affected by maternal age. The addition of maternal serum PAPP-A and PlGF to maternal factors improves the DR from 51 to 74% and 43 to 56%, at FPR of 10%, for PE requiring delivery before 34 and 37 weeks' gestation.

Q6. What is the ideal protocol for PE screening?

Draft Recommendation 6.1: *All pregnant women should be screened for preterm PE during early pregnancy by the first-trimester combined test that includes maternal risk factors, measurements of mean arterial pressure (MAP), serum placental growth factor (PlGF), and uterine artery pulsatility index (UTPI).*

All pregnant women should be screened for preterm PE during early pregnancy by the first-trimester combined test with maternal risk factors and biomarkers as a one-step procedure. The risk calculator is available free of charge at: *https://fetalmedicine.org/research/assess/preeclampsia*. FIGO encourages all countries and its member associations to adopt and promote strategies to ensure this. The best combined test is one that includes maternal risk factors, measurements of mean arterial pressure (MAP), serum placental growth factor (PlGF), and uterine artery pulsatility index (UTPI). A woman is considered high risk when the risk is 1 in 100 based on the first-trimester combined test with maternal risk factors, MAP, PlGF, and uterine artery PI.

Q7. What is the pragmatic protocol for PE screening?

Draft Recommendation 7.1: *In resource-limited settings, routine screening for preterm PE by maternal factors and MAP in all pregnancies and reserving measurements of PLGF and UTPI for a subgroup of the population, selected on the basis of the risk derived from screening by maternal factors and MAP, can be considered.*

Draft Recommendation 7.2: *Gestosis score is a maternal history based scoring system which can be used at all levels of healthcare facilities.*

Where resources are limited, routine screening for preterm PE by maternal factors and MAP in all pregnancies and reserving measurements of PLGF and UTPI for a subgroup of the population, selected on the basis of the risk derived from screening by maternal factors and MAP, can be considered. Implementation of guidelines is a constant challenge. The reality is that most developing countries around the world are unable to implement a first-trimester screening program for preterm PE based on the combined test. Recommendations that are rigid and impractical in real life settings are unlikely to be implemented and hence may produce little or no impact. On the other hand, pragmatic but less than ideal recommendations may produce significant impact due to more widespread implementation. In low- and middle-income countries where resources are limited, variations of the first trimester combined test can be considered but the baseline test is one that combines maternal risk factors with MAP. In the absence of one or two of the biomarker(s), risk calculation can still be done but the detection rates for preterm PE will be reduced, in turn leading to a reduction in the treatment effect size by aspirin prophylaxis but may make the treatment economically feasible.

Gestosis score: A careful history taken early in first trimester can warrant attention for effective prediction and prevention toward mothers "at risk" very early. This can be done by any healthcare worker by using HDP-gestosis score. It is an effective and feasible prediction policy.

Process of risk scoring: This score involves all the existing and emerging risk factors in the pregnant woman. Score 1, 2, and 3 is allotted to each clinical risk factor as per its severity in development of preeclampsia. With careful history and assessment of woman a total score is obtained time to time. When total score is ≥3; pregnant woman should be marked as "At risk for preeclampsia" **(Table 2)**.

Q8. What is the role of biochemical markers for prediction of preeclampsia in the second and third trimester?

Draft Recommendation 8.1: *The main aim of third trimester screening is to identify the subgroup that will develop severe PE requiring delivery within the subsequent 1–4 weeks.*

TABLE 2: Risk factor score.

Risk Factor	***Score***
Age >35 years	1
Age <19 years	1
Maternal anemia	1
Obesity (BMI >30)	1
Primigravida	1
Short duration of sperm exposure (cohabitation)	1
Woman born as small for gestational age	1
Family history of cardiovascular disease	1
Polycystic ovary syndrome	1
Inter pregnancy interval more than 7 years	1
Conceived with assisted reproductive (IVF/ICSI) treatment	1
MAP>85 mm of Hg	1
Chronic vascular disease (dyslipidemia)	1
Excessive weight gain during pregnancy	1
Maternal hypothyroidism	2
Family history of preeclampsia	2
Gestational diabetes mellitus	2
Obesity (BMI > 35 kg/m^2)	2
Multifetal pregnancy	2
Hypertensive disease during previous pregnancy	2
Pregestational diabetes mellitus	3
Chronic hypertension	3
Mental disorders	3
Inherited/acquired thrombophilia	3
Maternal chronic kidney disease	3
Autoimmune disease (SLE/APLAS/RA)	3
Pregnancy with assisted reproductive (OD or surrogacy) treatment	3

Good practice point: A Sflt-1/PIGF ratio of ≤33 rules out PE at the time of the test while a ratio of >85 at less than 32 weeks is suggestive of PE (rule in) and a value of >110 is suggestive of PE after 32 weeks (rule in).

Second trimester: The main value of the 22 weeks assessment is to identify first the high-risk group for development of early PE that would then require close monitoring for development of high blood pressure and proteinuria at 24–32 weeks and second the high-risk group for preterm PE that would require reassessment at around 32 weeks and on the basis of such assessment stratification into a high-risk group in need of close monitoring at 32–36 weeks and a low-risk group that would be reassessed at 36 weeks. Screening by maternal factors predicted 52, 47, and 37% of PE at <32, <37, and >37 week's gestation respectively at a false-positive rate of 10%. The respective values for combined screening with maternal factors and MAP, UTPI, and PLGF were 99, 85, and 46%. The performance was not improved by the addition of SFLT. Therefore, performance of screening for PE by maternal factors and biomarkers in the middle trimester is superior to taking a medical history.

Screening in third trimester: For early-onset PE, the first-trimester of pregnancy gives us an opportunity to do a good screening. However, late-onset PE still remains a challenge. The second stage screening at 30–33 weeks is required for predicting preeclampsia that aims at intensive close monitoring of these pregnancies by blood pressure measurements, proteinuria, and intensive fetal monitoring for growth restriction and warrants delivery at or after 34 weeks. This particular combines maternal characteristics and history, biochemical and biophysical markers at 30–33 week's gestation to estimate the risk of developing PE requiring delivery within selected intervals from the time of screening. MAP, UTPI, PLGF (pro-angiogenic), and SFLT (anti-angiogenic) at 30–34 week's gestation have been used to examine the potential improvement in performance of screening by maternal factors along with the addition of each biomarker and combinations of biomarkers. In pregnancies that developed PE, the values of MAP, UTPI, and SFLT were increased and PLGF was decreased.

Combined screening by maternal factors, MAP, UTPI, PLGF, and SFLT predicted 98% of preterm-PE and 49% of term-PE, at a false positive rate of 5%. The main aim of third trimester screening is to identify the subgroup that will develop severe PE requiring delivery within the subsequent 1–4 weeks. In such high-risk pregnancies, measurement of serum PlGF or soluble fms-like tyrosine kinase-1 (sFlt-1) to PlGF ratio is highly accurate in identifying the target group.

Sflt-1/PIGF ratio in diagnosis of early-onset preeclampsia:

- *Cut-off of ≤33:*
  - Ruled out PE at the time of the test
  - Sensitivity of 95.0% and a specificity of 94.0%
- *Cut-off of ≥85:*
  - Diagnosed PE
  - Sensitivity of 88.0% and a specificity of 99.5%.

Sflt-1/PIGF ratio in diagnosis of late-onset preeclampsia:

- *Cut-off of ≤33:*
  - Ruled out PE at the time of the test
  - Sensitivity of 89.6% and a specificity of 73.1%

- *Cut-off of ≥110:*
  - Diagnosed PE
  - Sensitivity of 58.2% and a specificity of 95.5%

BIBLIOGRAPHY

1. Ackerman CM, Platner MH, Spatz ES, et al. Severe cardiovascular morbidity in women with hypertensive diseases during delivery hospitalization. Am J Obstet Gynecol. 2019;220:582.e1-11.
2. American College of Obstetricians and Gynecologists. Committee opinion No. 638: first-trimester risk assessment for early-onset preeclampsia. Obstet Gynecol. 2015;126:e25-27.
3. Carr DB, Newton KM, Utzschneider KM, et al. Preeclampsia and risk of developing subsequent diabetes. Hypertens Preg. 2009;28:435-47.
4. Cunningham GC, Roberts JM, Lindheimer MD. The clinical spectrum of preeclampsia. In: Lindheimer MD, Roberts JM, Cunningham GC (Eds). Chesley's Hypertensive Disorders in Pregnancy. San Diego, CA: Elsevier; 2009.
5. Duley L. The global impact of preeclampsia and eclampsia. Semin Perinatol. 2009;33:130-7.
6. Fetal Medicine Foundation. Risk for preeclampsia. [online] Available from https://fetalmedicine.org/research/assess/preeclampsia/first-trimester. [Last accessed November, 2024]
7. FOGSI-GESTOSIS-ICOG. (2019). Hypertensive Disorders in Pregnancy (HDP) Good Clinical Practice Recommendations 2019. [online] Available from https://icogonline.org/wp-content/uploads/pdf/gcpr/hdp_fogsi_gestosis_icog_gcpr_2019.pdf. [Last accessed November, 2024]
8. Gallo D, Poon LC, Fernandez M, et al. Prediction of preeclampsia by mean arterial pressure at 11–13 and 20–24 week's gestation. Fetal Diagn Ther. 2014;36(1):28-37.
9. Gallo DM, Wright D, Casanova C, et al. Competing risks model in screening for preeclampsia by maternal factors and biomarkers at 19–24 weeks' gestation. Am J Obstet Gynecol. 2016;214:619.e1-17.
10. Granger JP, Alexander BT, Llinas MT, et al. Pathophysiology of hypertension during preeclampsia linking placental ischemia with endothelial dysfunction. Hypertension. 2001;38:718-22.
11. Gurgel Alves JA, Praciano de Sousa PC, Bezerra Maia E Holanda Moura S, et al. First-trimester maternal ophthalmic artery Doppler analysis for prediction of pre-eclampsia. Ultrasound Obstet Gynecol. 2014;44:411-8.
12. Hitti J, Sienas L, Walker S, et al. Contribution of hypertension to severe maternal morbidity. Am J Obstet Gynecol. 2018;219:405.e1-7.
13. Khaliq OP, Phoswa WN, Moodley J. The effectiveness of the Congo Red Dot paper test in hypertensive disorders of pregnancy: A systematic review and meta-analysis. Front Reprod Health. 2023;5:1120937.
14. Kuklina EV, Ayala C, Callaghan WM. Hypertensive disorders and severe obstetric morbidity in the United States. Obstet Gynecol. 2009;113:1299-306.
15. Magnussen EB, Vatten LJ, Smith GD, Romundstad PR. Hypertensive disorders in pregnancy and subsequently measured cardiovascular risk factors. Obstet Gynecol. 2009;114:961-70.

16. Matias DS, Costa RF, Matias BS, et al. Predictive value of ophthalmic artery Doppler velocimetry in relation to development of pre-eclampsia. Ultrasound Obstet Gynecol. 2014;44:419-26.
17. McDonald SD, Han Z, Walsh MW, et al. Kidney disease after preeclampsia: a systematic review and meta-analysis. Am J Kidney Dis. 2010;55:1026-39.
18. Meekins JW, Pijnenborg R, Hanssens M, et al. A study of placental bed spiral arteries and trophoblastic invasion in normal and severe preeclamptic pregnancies. BJOG. 1994;101:669-74.
19. Mol BWJ, Roberts CT, Thangaratinam S, et al. Preeclampsia. Lancet. 2016;387:999-1011.
20. Nagalla SR, Janaki V, Vijayalakshmi AR, et al. Glycosylated fibronectin point-of-care test for diagnosis of pre-eclampsia in a low-resource setting: a prospective Southeast Asian population study. BJOG. 2020;127(13):1687-94.
21. National Institute for Clinical Excellence. PLGF-based testing to help diagnose suspected preterm pre-eclampsia: diagnostics Guidance; 2022:1-27. [online] Available from http://www.nice.org.uk/guidance/dg49. [Last accessed November, 2024]
22. Plasencia W, Maiz N, Bonino S, et al. Uterine artery Doppler at 11 + 0 to 13 + 6 weeks in the prediction of pre-eclampsia. Ultrasound Obstet Gynecol. 2007;30:742-9.
23. Poon LC, Kametas NA, Chelemen T, et al. Maternal risk factors for hypertensive disorders in pregnancy: a multivariate approach. J Hum Hypertens. 2010;24:104-10.
24. Poon LC, Shennan A, Hyett JA, et al. The International Federation of Gynecology and Obstetrics (FIGO) initiative on pre-eclampsia: a pragmatic guide for first-trimester screening and prevention. Int J Gynaecol Obstet. 2019;145 Suppl 1(Suppl 1):1-33. Erratum in: Int J Gynaecol Obstet. 2019;146(3):390-1.
25. Praciano de Souza PC, Gurgel Alves JA, Bezerra Maia E Holanda Moura S, et al. Second trimester screening of preeclampsia using maternal characteristics and uterine and ophthalmic artery Doppler. Ultraschall Med. 2018;39:190-7.
26. Roberge S, Nicolaides KH, Demers S, et al. Prevention of perinatal death and adverse perinatal outcome using low-dose aspirin: a meta-analysis. Ultrasound Obstet Gynecol. 2013;41:491-9.
27. Roberge S, Villa P, Nicolaides K, et al. Early administration of low-dose aspirin for the prevention of preterm and term preeclampsia: a systematic review and meta-analysis. Fetal Diagn Ther. 2012;31:141-6.
28. Rolnik DL, Wright D, Poon LCY, et al. ASPRE trial: performance of screening for preterm pre-eclampsia. Ultrasound Obstet Gynecol. 2017;50(4):492-5. Erratum in: Ultrasound Obstet Gynecol. 2017;50(6):807.
29. Stevens W, Shih T, Incerti D, et al. Short term costs of preeclampsia to the United States health care system. Am J Obstet Gynecol. 2017;217:237-48.e16.
30. Tan MY, Syngelaki A, Poon LC, et al. Screening for pre-eclampsia by maternal factors and biomarkers at 11-13 weeks' gestation. Ultrasound Obstet Gynecol. 2018;52:186-95.
31. Tranquilli AL, Brown MA, Zeeman GG, et al. The definition of severe and early-onset preeclampsia. Statements from the International Society for the Study of Hypertension in Pregnancy (ISSHP). Pregnancy Hypertens. 2013;3:44-7.

32. Tsiakkas A, Saiid Y, Wright A, et al. Competing risks model in screening for preeclampsia by maternal factors and biomarkers at 30–34 weeks' gestation. Am J Obstet Gynecol. 2016;215(1):87.
33. Witlin GA, Saade GR, Mattar FM, et al. Predictors of neonatal outcome in women with severe preeclampsia or eclampsia between 24 and 33 week's gestation. Am J Obstet Gynecol. 2000;182:607-11.
34. Wright D, Syngelaki A, Bradbury I, et al. First-trimester screening for trisomies 21, 18 and 13 by ultrasound and biochemical testing. Fetal Diagn Ther. 2014;35:118-26.
35. Zeisler H, Llurba E, Chantraine F, et al. Predictive value of the sFlt-1: PlGF ratio in women with suspected preeclampsia. N Engl J Med. 2016;374(1):13-22.

CHAPTER 5

Preventive Strategies for Preeclampsia

Sujata Dalvi, Deepali Kapote

Q1. How can lifestyle changes prevent preeclampsia?

- Preconceptional weight reduction in overweight and obese patients or during interpregnancy intervals
- Regular physical activity of moderate intensity. Strict bed rest is not recommended for prevention of preeclampsia.
- Healthy, nutritious diet as advised for other pregnant women
- Removal/reduction of stress or exertion should be advised.

Summary of evidence: Strict bed rest for pregnant women at risk of hypertension is not advised as per WHO recommendations. Such patients at risk of pre-eclampsia are given same lifestyle advice as healthy pregnant women as mentioned in NICE guidelines 133.

Do not advise rest or dietary salt restriction for pregnant women to prevent gestational hypertension, preeclampsia, or its complications as per WHO and NICE guidelines 133.

As per a systematic review of meta-analysis, intervention in the form of exercise reduced the risk of preeclampsia in patients with raised BMI.

Q2. What is the role, dosage, and duration of aspirin in prevention of preeclampsia?

- Aspirin irreversibly inactivates the cyclooxygenase-1 enzyme, suppressing the production of prostaglandins and thromboxane and inhibiting inflammation and platelet aggregation.
- This helps in the second wave of villous invasion and decreases the vascular resistance in the placental blood vessels, thus preventing preeclampsia.
- Tablet Aspirin 75–150 mg (according to BMI) once daily to be started in patients with risk factors as soon as pregnancy is confirmed and continued till delivery.

Summary of evidence: Recommendations for low-dose aspirin for prevention of preeclampsia.

Organization and dose recommendation:

- *USPSTF (2021):* 81 mg daily after 12 weeks of gestation with any high-risk condition or more than 1 moderate-risk condition

- *ACOG or SMFM (2021):* 81 mg daily between 12 and 28 weeks of gestation (ideally by 16 weeks) with any high-risk conditions or more than 1 moderate-risk condition
- *WHO:* 75 mg daily before 20 weeks of gestation with any high-risk condition
- *NICE (2019):* 75–150 mg daily after 12 weeks of gestation with any high-risk condition

(ACOG: American College of Obstetricians and Gynecologists; NICE: National Institute for Health and Care Excellence; SMFM: Society for Maternal-Fetal Medicine; USPSTF: United States Preventative Services Task Force; WHO: World Health Organization)

As per NICE guidelines 133, advise pregnant women to take 75–150 mg of aspirin daily from 12 weeks until the birth of the baby as follows:

At least 1 high-risk factor	*At least 2 moderate-risk factors*
Hypertensive disease during a previous pregnancy	Nulliparity
Chronic kidney disease	Age 40 years or older
Autoimmune disease such as systemic lupus erythematosus or antiphospholipid syndrome	Pregnancy interval of more than 10 years
Type 1 or type 2 diabetes	Body mass index (BMI) of 35 kg/m^2 or more at first visit
Chronic hypertension	Family history of pre-eclampsia
	Multi fetal pregnancy

Q3. What is the role of calcium, vitamin D_3, and folic acid supplementation in prevention of preeclampsia?

- Calcium supplementation of at least 1 g daily from mid-pregnancy (20 weeks) is associated with reduction in risk of preeclampsia if the recommended daily allowance of 1 g/day is not met through nutrition.
- Vitamin D_3 supplementation 400 IU daily should be provided as per deficiency status. There is negative association between development of preeclampsia, small for gestational age fetus, preterm birth, and vitamin D deficiency.
- Folic acid has no separate role than routine antenatal prophylaxis for preeclampsia prevention.

Summary of evidence: As per WHO recommendations, calcium supplementation during pregnancy in areas where calcium intake is low (<900 mg/day). A meta-analysis showed the risk reduction for preeclampsia was statistically significant in patients with low baseline calcium intake.

Also, vitamin D supplementation during pregnancy is not recommended as low-quality studies are available.

The body of data does not indicate a consistent decreased or increased risk for hypertensive disorders of pregnancy with low or high dose of folic acid. It is still recommended in preconceptional counseling.

Q4. What is the role of micronutrient supplementation like antioxidant (vitamin C and E), magnesium, omega 3 fatty acid, fish oils, L-arginine, coenzyme Q10, and progesterone supplementation in the prevention of preeclampsia?

- Antioxidants like vitamin C and E may have some role but there are no definite studies for routine use of antioxidants in pregnancy.
- Magnesium supplementation is useful for secondary prevention of preeclampsia but its role in primary prevention is not well established.
- Evidence of routine use of L-arginine, omega 3 fatty acid, co-enzyme Q10 in prevention of preeclampsia is limited, hence not recommended.
- Progesterone supplementation is advisable.

Summary of evidence: As per WHO recommendations, individual or combined vitamin C and vitamin E supplementation is not to be prescribed for prevention of preeclampsia although it may be useful in other conditions.

Do not recommend the following supplements solely with the aim of preventing hypertensive disorders during pregnancy: Magnesium, folic acid, antioxidants (vitamins C and E), fish oils or algal oils, garlic as mentioned in NICE guidelines 133.

Due to limited availability of data on use of micronutrient supplementation in use of preeclampsia prevention, their use is not recommended.

5. What are the prospects of using low-molecular weight heparin, statins (pravastatin), metformin, nitric oxide donors and diuretics in patients with high risk of preeclampsia?

- Low-molecular weight heparin combined with aspirin is helpful in patients of inherited thrombophilias only. Limited data on combined use of anticoagulants and aspirin for routine prevention of preeclampsia.
- Pravastatin and metformin is not recommended in such cases.
- Patients at high risk of preeclampsia have shown little or no benefit from use of nitric oxide donors (vasodilators) and diuretics.

Summary of evidence: Available data do not conclusively support use of low-molecular weight heparin prophylaxis in addition to low-dose aspirin to reduce the risk of preeclampsia or its sequelae, although these data are not definitive, and there are methodologic concerns with the published trials.

Pravastatin has promising effects but evidence is limited to a few randomized control trials only.

Similar to statins, metformin has been shown to alter angiogenic imbalance by decreasing sFlt-1 and soluble endoglin. A meta-analysis of studies in high-risk women with insulin resistance did not show a reduction in preeclampsia compared with placebo or control.

As per NICE guidelines 133, use of nitric oxide donors, diuretics is not recommended.

Use of diuretics, particularly thiazides, for prevention of preeclampsia and its complications is not advised as per WHO recommendations.

Q6. How can decision of age at first pregnancy, pregnancy interval, and change of paternity prevent preeclampsia?

- Recommending to get pregnant at ages 20–24; avoiding pregnancy under the age of 20 and over the age of 35; avoiding intervals of 10 years or higher between pregnancies.
- Usage of donor oocytes/semen has shown an increased incidence of preeclampsia.

Q7. How can secondary prevention of preeclampsia be done?

- Screening of all patients on routine antenatal visits.
- Early initiation of treatment with antihypertensives (BP 140/90)
- High degree of suspicion for complications and aggressive monitoring.
- Continuation of pregnancy with pre-eclampsia with close monitoring
- Injection $MgSO_4$ for impending eclampsia.
- Stabilization and prompt referral to higher center under supervision.

Summary of recommendations: Antihypertensive drugs for pregnant women with BP 140/90 are recommended by CHIPS trial.

Regular monitoring of blood pressure and urinary protein can help in early diagnosis and prevention of complications is recommended by all guidelines.

Q8. Can placental growth factor assessment, fetal biomarkers (β-HCG, PAPP-A, AFP), serum uric acid levels, and 2nd trimester Doppler studies be used for secondary prevention of preeclampsia?

- These biomarkers are of theoretical and retrospective value
- Placental growth factor is used to assess disease progression
- Serum β-HCG and alpha-fetoprotein may be raised and PAPP-A is observed to fall in patients of preeclampsia.
- Serum uric acid levels are found to be raised in patients of preeclampsia.
- Uterine artery Doppler in second trimester is a useful tool for prediction and secondary prevention of pre-eclampsia.

Summary of evidence: Biochemical markers like placental growth factor, β-hCG, PAPP-A, alpha fetoprotein, and serum uric acid levels can be used for early prediction as per ACOG guidelines but their usage is limited by a number of factors like availability, cost-effectiveness, and lack of sensitivity and positive predictive value.

Q9. What is the correlation between treatment of chronic diseases like overt diabetes, renal dysfunction, SLE, APS, vascular disease, and preeclampsia risk reduction?

- Type 2 diabetes mellitus, chronic renal disease, systemic lupus erythematosus with or without antiphospholipid antibody syndrome, and vascular diseases are associated with increased of development of preeclampsia due to decreased uteroplacental blood flow.
- Optimizing disease condition before conception and screening of preeclampsia is necessary for early diagnosis and prompt management and successful outcomes.

Summary of evidence: As per NICE guidelines 133, control of overt diabetes and chronic diseases is necessary to prevent preeclampsia as there is positive correlation between them.

Q10. What is the role of gestosis score in prediction and prevention of preeclampsia?

- A scoring system that takes into account both established and newly recognized factors that are linked to the causation of gestational hypertension.
- After conducting a thorough assessment and detailed medical histories, a cumulative score is determined for each participant.
- Gestosis score is a novel early marker for prediction of the development of PE allowing for a prompt management for the patients, thereby curbing the adverse consequences.
- As per one Indian study, gestosis score of 3 or more has:
  - Diagnostic accuracy (95.35%) for predicting the development of preeclampsia (PE)
  - *Sensitivity:* 83.1%
  - *Specificity:* 97.51%
  - *PPV:* 85.51%
  - *NPV:* 97.03%, indicating the probability of a negative result.

Gestosis score 1	*Gestosis score 2*	*Gestosis score 3*
Age older than 35 years	Maternal hypothyroidism	Pregestational diabetes mellitus
Age younger than 19 years	Hypertensive disease during previous pregnancy	Chronic hypertension

Contd...

Contd...

Gestosis score 1	***Gestosis score 2***	***Gestosis score 3***
Maternal anemia	Family history of preeclampsia	Mental disorders
Obesity (BMI >30)	Gestational diabetes mellitus	Inherited/acquired thrombophilia
Primigravida	Obesity (BMI >35 kg/m^2)	Maternal chronic kidney disease
Short duration of sperm exposure (cohabitation)	Multifetal pregnancy	Autoimmune disease (SLE/APLAS/RA)
Woman born as small for gestational age		Pregnancy with assisted reproductive (OD or surrogacy) treatment
Family history of cardiovascular disease		
Polycystic ovary syndrome		
Inter pregnancy interval more than 7 years		
Conceived with assisted reproductive (IVF/ICSI) treatment		
MAP >85 mm of Hg		
Chronic vascular disease (dyslipidemia)		
Excessive weight gain during pregnancy		

BIBLIOGRAPHY

1. American College of Obstetricians and Gynaecologists. Hypertension in pregnancy. Report of the American College of Obstetricians and Gynecologists' Task Force on Hypertension in Pregnancy. Obstet Gynecol. 2013;122(5):1122-31.
2. Danielli M, Gillies C, Thomas RC, et al. Effects of Supervised Exercise on the Development of Hypertensive Disorders of Pregnancy: A Systematic Review and Meta-Analysis. J Clin Med. 2022;11(3):793.
3. Gupta M, Yadav P, Yaqoob F. A Prospective Study to Determine the Predictive Ability of HDP-Gestosis Score for the Development of Pre-eclampsia. J Obstet Gynaecol India. 2022;72(6):485-491.
4. Markham K, Funai EF. Pregnancy-related hypertension. In: Creasy RK, Resnik R, Iams JD (Eds). Creasy and Resnik's Maternal-Fetal Medicine, 7th edition. Philadelphia: Elsevier; 2015. pp. 756-81.
5. NICE Guidelines NG 133. (2019). Guidelines on delivery, planning, including the use of Caesarean section.
6. Woo Kinshella ML, Sarr C, Sandhu A, et al. Calcium for pre-eclampsia prevention: A systematic review and network meta-analysis to guide personalised antenatal care. BJOG. 2022;129(11):1833-43.
7. World Health Organization. WHO recommendations for prevention and treatment of preeclampsia and eclampsia. Geneva: World Health Organization; 2013.

CHAPTER 6

Clinical Features of Preeclampsia

Munjal Pandya, Ashish Varma

Q1. What are the typical presenting features of preeclampsia?

Draft recommendations:

- *One-third of cases are nulliparous:*
    - *High-risk factors:* Overweight/obesity/prior preeclampsia/multifetal pregnancy/chronic hypertension/preexisting diabetes/chronic kidney disease increases the chances of developing preeclampsia. Sudden weight gain over 1–2 days or more than 2 pounds (0.9 kg) a week
- Early-onset preeclampsia (<34 weeks of gestation) develops in <10% of patients out of total pre-eclampsia. Very rarely, it can develop at 20–22 weeks as well.
- Approximately 85% of patients develop new-onset hypertension and proteinuria in late third trimester (>34 weeks of gestation) and sometimes in labor.
- Postpartum preeclampsia is seen in 5% total cases of preexisting eclampsia within 48 hour of delivery/cesarean section.
- The presenting features in form of hypertension, proteinuria, and other clinical manifestation are highly variable.

Summary of evidence: As per publication on clinical risk factors by Bartsch et al., the risk factors along with maternal hypertension would indicate presence of preeclampsia with higher probability. As per literature by Sibai BM, Cunningham FG, Yancey LM, Matthys LA, et al., majority of patients present with late preeclampsia. While very few cases present with early onset preeclampsia and very rarely they present with postpartum preeclampsia. The clinical features may vary and one or more may be present in cases presenting as preeclampsia.

Q2. What are the blood pressure parameters and symptoms of preeclampsia?

Draft recommendations:

- At least 25% of patients with preeclampsia develop severe hypertension (≥160/110 mm Hg) with one or more of the following presenting symptoms characterizing severe disease:
    - Persistent or severe headache

- Visual abnormalities
- Epigastric pain
- Altered mental conscious level
- Breathing difficulties

Summary of evidence: Patients with preeclampsia will develop severe hypertension in 1/4th of the cases. As per various reviews, variable symptoms will be present depending upon the organs/system affected. Development of hypertensive retinopathy and ophthalmic changes will lead to visual symptoms and headache. Stretching of Glisson's capsule will lead to severe epigastric pain.

Q3. What are the rare and atypical features of preeclampsia?

Draft recommendations:

- *Onset <20 weeks:* Very rarely patients will present with preeclampsia <20 weeks complete or partial hydatidiform mole and/or antiphospholipid syndrome.
- *Postpartum pre-eclampsia:* In at least 5% of total preeclampsia cases, the presenting features are seen in postpartum phase; headache being the most common symptom presenting in 70% of cases of preeclampsia. At least 20–30% of cases will present with breathing difficulties.
- Atypical features in the form of mild headaches with intermittent hypertension are seemingly few of the cases.
- Patients may present with preeclampsia even in absence of presenting symptoms.

Summary of evidence: Publication by Redman EK, Al Safii Z Fileting, et al. showed that headache was the most common symptoms in case of postpartum pre-eclampsia. Various studies by Sibai M et al. showed that atypical presentation of headache can be differentiated from other diseases like PRES or impending stroke. Punctuations by AL Safi Z, Filetti, LC Bigelow, et al. showed that delayed postpartum preeclampsia had similar risk factors of typical preeclampsia while some of the cases did not show any risk factors.

Q4. What are the severe features associated with a typical case of preeclampsia?

Draft recommendations:

- Severe hypertension (>160/110 mm Hg) on 2 occasions more than 4 hours apart.
- *Central nervous system symptoms:* New-onset visual/cerebral symptoms; i.e., scotomata, photopsia, cortical blindness, retinal vasospasm, and/or severe headache not relatively by routine medication of headache.

- *Symptoms related to hepatic system:* Altered liver enzyme levels (more than twice upper limit of normal range of transaminases levels) and/or severe epigastric pain not responding to medication
- Thrombocytopenia (platelet <100,000/microliter)
- *Symptoms related to renal system:* Serum creatinine >1.1 mg/dL
- Pulmonary edema

Summary of evidence: According to the American College of Obstetrics and Gyneclogy Practice Bulletin 222 Gestational Hypertension in Pregnancy, typical cases of preeclampsia will present with one or more of the above symptoms.

Q5. Can features of severe preeclampsia occur without hypertension?

Draft recommendations: It is very uncommon to have severe features of preeclampsia without hypertension but can occur in 15% of patients with HELLP or eclampsia. In this cases, the blood pressure may rise but does not reach the diagnostic limits of preeclampsia.

Summary of evidence: According to Zeeman GG, 15% of cases of HELLP may present with features of severe preeclampsia without hypertension.

Q6. Can isolated hypertension without severe features of pre-eclampsia develop severe features as the pregnancy advances?

Draft recommendations:

- Usually gestational hypertension is the term used for new-onset mild hypertension without features of preeclampsia.
- Approximately 50% patients will develop preeclampsia as the pregnancy advances.

Summary of evidence: According to Melvin et al., gestational hypertension in 50% of cases will develop preeclampsia needing monitoring.

Q7. Is it important to diagnose isolated proteinuria?

Draft recommendations:

- Isolated gestational proteinuria may occur in absence of symptoms of preeclampsia.
- At least 20–22% of cases may develop preeclampsia.
- Chronic renal disease should be ruled it in patients presenting isolated proteinuria.

Summary of evidence: According to Shinar S, et al., 13 patients out of 95 pregnant females with new-onset isolated proteinuria developed antepartum/intrapartum preeclampsia. 8 patients of those 95 developed postpartum preeclampsia.

BIBLIOGRAPHY

1. Al-Safi Z, Imudia AN, Filetti LC, et al. Delayed postpartum preeclampsia and eclampsia: demographics, clinical course, and complications. Obstet Gynecol. 2011;118:1102.
2. Bakhru A, Atlas RO. A case of postpartum cerebral angiitis and review of the literature. Arch Gynecol Obstet. 2011;283:663.
3. Bartsch E, Medcalf KE, Park AL, et al. Clinical risk factors for pre-eclampsia determined in early pregnancy: systematic review and meta-analysis of large cohort studies. BMJ. 2016;353:i1753.
4. Bigelow CA, Pereira GA, Warmsley A, et al. Risk factors for new-onset late postpartum preeclampsia in women without a history of preeclampsia. Am J Obstet Gynecol. 2014;210:338.e1.
5. Filetti LC, Imudia AN, Al-Safi Z, et al. New onset delayed postpartum preeclampsia: different disorders? J Matern Fetal Neonatal Med. 2012;25:957.
6. Macdonald-Wallis C, Lawlor DA, Heron J, et al. Relationships of risk factors for pre-eclampsia with patterns of occurrence of isolated gestational proteinuria during normal term pregnancy. PLoS One. 2011;6:e22115.
7. Redman EK, Hauspurg A, Hubel CA, et al. Clinical Course, Associated Factors, and Blood Pressure Profile of Delayed-Onset Postpartum Preeclampsia. Obstet Gynecol. 2019;134:995.
8. Shinar S, Asher-Landsberg J, Schwartz A, et al. Isolated proteinuria is a risk factor for pre-eclampsia: a retrospective analysis of the maternal and neonatal outcomes in women presenting with isolated gestational proteinuria. J Perinatol. 2016;36:25.
9. Sibai BM. Etiology and management of postpartum hypertension-preeclampsia. Am J Obstet Gynecol. 2012;206:470.
10. Zeeman GG. Neurologic complications of pre-eclampsia. Semin Perinatol. 2009;33:166.

CHAPTER 7

Maternal Evaluation in Preeclampsia

Uma Singh

Q1. What are various clinical and laboratory parameters in maternal evaluation of preeclampsia?

Draft recommendations:

- Maternal evaluation for preeclampsia must include both clinical and laboratory parameters. Clinical evaluation includes blood pressure monitoring which should be done four hourly.
- Blood pressure measurement is the most important clinical test to diagnostic HDP.
- BP assessment is to be done with utmost care and proper technique. Mercury manometer periodically standardized is the ideal equipment to be used. Cuff size is important specially in patients with high BMI. Patient should be comfortable with empty bladder, should not have smoked or chewed tobacco for 1 hour prior.
- The position of the pregnant mother, especially after 20 weeks of gestation should be either in the sitting position or left lateral position with the zero level at the level of the heart. Any forearm left/right can be used to tie the cuff of the appropriate size snuggly.
- In absence of mercury manometer, calibrated aneroid equipment may be used. However, mercury sphygmomanometer is the gold standard. Calibration is required only for aneroid or electronic BP instruments.
- Strict vigilance for symptoms like headache, blurring of vision, epigastric pain, excessive weight gain, pedal edema is of utmost importance for evaluation of assessment of severity of preeclampsia. Feeling of ill-being of patient, difficulty in breathing, brisk tendon reflexes, uncontrolled hypertension, altered consciousness are other symptoms which warrant prompt management.
- Required laboratory investigations are hemoglobin, hematocrit, platelet count, 24 hours urine protein, serum transaminases (SGOT, SGPT), serum albumin, serum creatinine, serum LDH, serum uric acid, peripheral blood smear and coagulation profile.
- Coagulation profile and serum electrolytes are needed in severe cases.
- ACOG currently recommends diagnosing preeclampsia with either a 24-hour value or a protein creatinine ratio in a single voided urine. However, A spot urine protein creatinine ratio >0.3 mg/dL has been

shown to meet or exceed 300 mg protein on a 24 hours urine. So, 24-hour urine protein is replaced by spot urine protein creatinine ratio as it is cumbersome.

- Fundoscopy may be required to differentiate chronic and new onset disease and to diagnose papilledema/hemorrhages as these have ominous prognosis.

Q2. What is diagnostic accuracy of these parameters?

Draft recommendations:

- Test performance for urine dipstick testing is poor and variable.
- In a systematic review, protein creatinine ratio was evaluated in 1516 pregnant women in twelve studies. The range of test sensitivity was from 65% (95% CI not calculable) to 96% (95% CI, 88–99%).
- Optimal P/C ratio for detection of urine protein excretion of 300 mg/day was identified as 0.45 mg/mg with a sensitivity and specificity of 74.4% and 94.2%, respectively.
- Saleem FR et al. have shown that LDH has sensitivity of 50%, specificity of 80%, a positive predictive value of 70% and a negative predictive value of 61.54% (cut-off: 525 IU/L) in preeclampsia.
- Uric acid at a cut-off point ≥1.5 had a very low positive predictive value. However, it was found to have high negative predictive value of 99.5% for preeclampsia.

Q3. What is significance of proteinuria in pregnancy in preeclampsia?

Draft recommendations:

- Proteinuria is sufficient but not necessary for the diagnosis of preeclampsia as per latest guidelines.
- Proteinuria during pregnancy is defined when >300 mg/24 hours, protein is present or a urine protein-to-creatinine ratio of at least 0.3.
- However, excess protein secretion is not found to be a causative factor for poor maternal and neonatal outcome. Rather poor maternal and neonatal outcomes is found to be associated in the presence of end organ damage and severity of blood pressure. That is why, monitoring proteinuria is not recommended.

Q4. What should be frequency of laboratory evaluation?

Draft recommendations:

- Maternal evaluation should include review of symptomatology associated with severe preeclampsia, blood pressure measurement, and weekly laboratory testing (platelet count, serum creatinine, and liver transaminases).

- The recommendation for weekly laboratory testing is based on expert opinion, with the goal of early detection of severe preeclampsia and associated end-organ damage.

Q5. What is role of expectant management in severe preeclampsia?

Draft recommendations:

- The aim of delaying delivery is to gain more time for the premature fetus so that neonatal morbidity and mortality can be reduced from preterm birth but with strict maternofetal monitoring to avoid serious maternal or fetal complications from disease progression.
- Persistent severe hypertension unresponsive to antihypertensive therapy, symptoms which indicate for severe disease like severe persistent headache which is new onset and not responding to acetaminophen, blurring of vision, epigastric pain or motor deficit, altered sensorium, pulmonary edema, renal failure, stroke or laboratory abnormalities, such as:
    - Aminotransferases increasing over 6–12 hours and reaching levels twice the upper limit of normal
    - Progressive decrease in platelet count to <100,000 cells/μL
    - Coagulopathy
    - New or worsening renal dysfunction [serum creatinine >1.1 mg/dL (97 micromol/L) or twice baseline]
- Two trials reported significant prolongation of pregnancy and improvement in neonatal outcome with expectant management, with no increase in the rate of maternal complications if there is no contraindication for prolongation. But conservative management to be done only at tertiary care level, i.e., level 3 hospital.
- Prompt delivery for all patients with preeclampsia with severe features who have reached ≥34 weeks of gestation is advocated.

Research gap:

- There is emerging literature suggesting role of angiogenic factors (sFlt-1, PlGF) for prediction of adverse outcomes in preeclampsia by combining them with other clinical and laboratory parameters.
- In the PRediction of short-term Outcome in preGNant wOmen with Suspected preeclampsIa Study (PROGNOSIS), an sFlt-1/PlGF ratio cut-off of ≤ 38 was validated and it was found that it ruled out preeclampsia within 1 week [negative predictive value [NPV] 99.3%] or 4 weeks (NPV 94.3%), while ratio values above 38 ruled in preeclampsia within 4 weeks [positive predictive value (PPV) > 36%].
- Women with a ratio test result of 38–85 will require increased surveillance, mostly as outpatients, with an initial retest after 1–2 weeks to assess

whether there has been a change in the markers for prediction of development of preeclampsia.

- In the INSPIRE trial ratio cut-off value of ≥ 85 has shown positive predictive value of 71.7% to rule in preeclampsia in next 4 weeks. In the Rule Out Pre-Eclampsia (ROPE) study, women with suspected preeclampsia presenting at <34 weeks of gestation, sFlt-1/PlGF ratio > 85 had PPV of 74% for development of severe preeclampsia within two weeks. Gestational age related cut offs had been given in a study by Verlohren et al. which included 1,149 patients. They found that ratios of > 85 (20–33 + 6 weeks) and > 110 (34 weeks to delivery) strongly associated with the development of preeclampsia.
- The sFlt-1/PlGF ratio is a test that can help rule out pre-eclampsia, detect its progression, and improve clinical precision. It can also reduce the time it takes to diagnose pre-eclampsia and lower the incidence of adverse maternal outcomes.
- Studies have shown limited value of repeat PlGF-based testing in women with suspected preterm preeclampsia. With an estimated 5% of women globally experiencing preterm pregnancy hypertension, of 140 million births, there is now a clear evidence base for implementation of initial PlGF-based testing, but without the necessity of higher costs associated with repeat PlGF-based testing.
- Currently, the ratio can be used to estimate the expected time to delivery only as an adjunct to all the clinical information available for the patient, ranging from BP, laboratory findings, ultrasound, Doppler scans and symptoms—the sFlt-1/PlGF ratio is an additional data point and can be regarded as adjunct to clinical care when making delivery decisions.
- There are some emerging evidences that serum uric acid level may be useful in 2nd and 3rd trimester of pregnancy. It along with biochemical and USG markers may have prognostic value if the FGR has occurred due to preeclampsia pathology and other causes are not responsible for it. More studies are required to establish his correlation.

BIBLIOGRAPHY

1. American College of Obstetricians and Gynaecologists. Hypertension in pregnancy. Report of the American College of Obstetricians and Gynecologists' Task Force on Hypertension in Pregnancy. Obstet Gynecol. 2013;122(5):1122-31.
2. Barton JR, Istwan NB, Rhea D, et al. Cost-savings analysis of an outpatient management program for women with pregnancy-related hypertensive conditions. Dis Manag. 2006;9(04):236-41.
3. Cerdeira AS, O'Sullivan J, Ohuma EO, et al. Performance of soluble fms-like tyrosine kinase-1-to-placental growth factor ratio of ≥85 for ruling in preeclampsia within 4 weeks. Am J Obstet Gynecol. 2021;224(3):322-3.

4. Corominas AI, Medina Y, Balconi S, et al. Assessing the role of uric acid as a predictor of preeclampsia. Front Physiol. 2022;12:785219.
5. Demirci O, Kumru P, Arınkan A, et al. Spot protein/creatinine ratio in preeclampsia as an alternative for 24-hour urine protein. Balkan Med J. 2015;32(1):51-5.
6. Fishel Bartal M, Lindheimer MD, Sibai BM. Proteinuria during pregnancy: definition, pathophysiology, methodology, and clinical significance. Am J Obstet Gynecol. 2022;226(2S):S819-S834.
7. Henderson JT, Thompson JH, Burda BU, et al. Preeclampsia Screening: Evidence Report and Systematic Review for the US Preventive Services Task Force. JAMA. 2017;317(16):1668-83.
8. Hurrell A, Webster L, Sparkes J, et al. Repeat placental growth factor-based testing in women with suspected preterm pre-eclampsia (PARROT-2): a multicentre, parallel-group, superiority, randomised controlled trial. Lancet. 2024;403(10427):619-31.
9. Odendaal HJ, Pattinson RC, Bam R, et al. Aggressive or expectant management for patients with severe preeclampsia between 28–34 weeks' gestation: a randomized controlled trial. Obstet Gynecol. 1990;76:1070.
10. Rana S, Salahuddin S, Mueller A, et al. Angiogenic biomarkers in triage and risk for preeclampsia with severe features. Pregnancy Hypertens. 2018;13:100-6.
11. Saleem FR, Chandru S, Biswas M. Evaluation of total LDH and its isoenzymes as markers in preeclampsia. J Med Biochem. 2020;39(3):392-8.
12. Sibai BM, Mercer BM, Schiff E, et al. Aggressive versus expectant management of severe preeclampsia at 28 to 32 weeks' gestation: a randomized controlled trial. Am J Obstet Gynecol. 1994;171:818.
13. Verdonk K, Niemeijer IC, Hop WC, et al. Variation of urinary protein to creatinine ratio during the day in women with suspected pre-eclampsia. BJOG. 2014;121(13):1660-5.
14. Verlohren S, Herraiz I, Lapaire O, et al New gestational phase-specific cutoff values for the use of the soluble fms-like tyrosine kinase-1/placental growth factor ratio as a diagnostic test for preeclampsia. Hypertension. 2014;63(2):346-52.
15. Wagner LK. Diagnosis and management of preeclampsia. Am Fam Physician. 2004;70(12):2317-24.
16. Wheeler TL 2nd, Blackhurst DW, Dellinger EH, et al. Usage of spot urine protein to creatinine ratios in the evaluation of preeclampsia. Am J Obstet Gynecol. 2007;196(5):e461-4.
17. Young RA, Buchanan RJ, Kinch RA. Use of the protein/creatinine ratio of a single voided urine specimen in the evaluation of suspected pregnancy-induced hypertension. J Fam Pract. 1996;42(4):385-9.
18. Zeisler H, Llurba E, Chantraine F, et al. Predictive value of the sFlt-1: PlGF ratio in women with suspected preeclampsia. N Engl J Med. 2016;374(1):13-22.

CHAPTER 8

Therapeutics in Preeclampsia

Ritu Khanna, Vidya Thobbi

8.1 HYPERTENSIVE DISORDERS IN PREGNANCY

Ritu Khanna

KEY QUESTIONS

1. Which antihypertensive drugs are used in preeclampsia?
2. When to start antihypertensive drugs in pregnancy?
3. Which antihypertensives drugs are contraindicated in pregnancy?
4. What drugs are used to manage hypertensive crisis in pregnancy?
5. What are the adverse effects of antihypertensive drugs used in preeclampsia?

Q1. Which antihypertensive drugs are used in preeclampsia?

Draft recommendations:

1. Antihypertensives drugs that are considered safe to take during pregnancy include:
   - *Labetalol:* A combined alpha- and beta-blocker (*high level of evidence*)
   - It is now available as 200 mg tablets as well. Maximum recommended dose is 2,400 mg in 3 or 4 divided doses.
   - *Nifedipine:* A calcium-channel blocker *(high level of evidence)*, available as standard oral form, nifedipine retard tablet, and controlled release form (CR). Controlled-release form is unavailable in India, recently available in the market in Japan.
   - Nifedipine controlled-release (CR or extended release—ER) is a long-acting, once-daily medication. It features a polymer matrix that includes a slow-release outer coat and a fast-release internal core. The outer layer dissolves at a slower rate compared to the inner layer, contributing to a prolonged release of the drug. This formulation allows for relatively stable plasma concentrations of nifedipine over a 24-hour period. Nifedipine CR is expected to induce less activation of the sympathetic nervous system compared to the nifedipine retard formulation.
   - Short-acting nifedipine is associated with abrupt decreases in systemic arterial blood pressure and greater reflex increases in activity of the sympathetic nervous system due to which it should be avoided in patients with cardiovascular disease.

- Sublingual route of nifedipine is not recommended and should be avoided as it may cause sudden precipitous fall in blood pressure (maternal hypotension) and fetal distress.
- *Nicardipine:* A nicardipine, a dihydropyridine calcium-channel blocker. It can be effectively used as an oral form as well as an intravenous formulation for treating severe and non-severe hypertension in pregnancy based on its high success rate and acceptable safety profile. Can be a first-line treatment in women with severe hypertension in pregnancy.
- *Hydralazine:* Oral hydralazine can be an effective option for managing nonsevere hypertension during pregnancy, but it should be used with caution and under close monitoring. *(Moderate level of evidence)*
- Nifedipine and hydralazine can cause reflex tachycardia. They are not recommended to be used in patients with heart rate above 100/min. Labetalol is an appropriate drug in such patients.
- Labetalol should be avoided in patients with bradycardia (heart rate <60 bpm, asthma and in congestive cardiac failure). Nifedipine is the drug of choice in such cases *as per FOGSI-GCPR.*
- *Methyldopa:* A central nervous system alpha-agonist, category B drug, currently unavailable in India.

They are based on observational data and meta-analyses of clinical trials and years of clinical practice.

2. Antihypertensive drugs that are selectively used in pregnancy:
   - *Diazoxide:* A potassium channel activator that causes vasodilation and reduces blood pressure (*Level of Evidence: Low*)
   - *Amlodipine:* Although there is not much information on its safety (*Level of Evidence: Low to Moderate*)

Summary of evidence: Hypertension in pregnancy is associated with an increased risk of fetal morbidity and mortality, as well as maternal sequelae including stroke, pulmonary edema, and death. Therefore, antihypertensive medications are often used to lower BP, prolong the pregnancy, and improve maternal and neonatal health outcomes.

CHAP (Chronic Hypertension and Pregnancy) Trial found that treating women with mild chronic hypertension during pregnancy to a BP target of <140/90 mm Hg was associated with better pregnancy outcomes compared to a strategy of reserving treatment only for those with severe hypertension. ACOG now recommends utilizing 140/90 mm Hg as the threshold for initiation or titration of medical therapy for chronic hypertension in pregnancy.

Research gaps: Future studies comparing medication effectiveness in pregnant patients with distinct hypertensive disorders (chronic hypertension/preeclampsia/gestational hypertension) are needed.

According to NCBI, there is a lack of clinical trial evidence that compares the safety and efficacy of antihypertensive drugs during pregnancy. This means that there are no specific guidelines for selecting and dosing medications.

Due to the various physiologic changes experienced during pregnancy, pregnancy-associated changes in pharmacokinetics and pharmacodynamics of many drugs, including antihypertensive medications, occur in pregnant individuals. Hence initial selection and dosing strategies remain unclear due to a lack of clinical evidence comparing the safety and effectiveness of different treatment strategies.

Q2. When to start antihypertensive drugs in pregnancy?

Draft recommendations:

Various Society Recommendations:

- Determining the optimal BP threshold in pregnancy for antihypertensive treatment and therapeutic targets requires a balance between the prevention of maternal hypertensive complications and the avoidance of fetal risks *[Level of Evidence: High (ACOG and NICE)]*
- Personalization of therapy, by giving special attention to other risk factors related to hypertension-related adverse outcomes (such as preexisting heart or kidney disease, obesity, and Black race), is a rational approach *[Level of Evidence: High (AHA and ACC)]*
- As per the recent CHAP (Chronic Hypertension in Pregnancy) trial found that treating women with mild chronic hypertension during pregnancy to a BP target<140/90 mm Hg was associated with better pregnancy outcomes compared to a strategy of reserving treatment only for those with severe hypertension.
- *Chronic hypertension:* Antihypertensive medications should be initiated if the woman has chronic hypertension and her blood pressure is persistently above 140/90 mm Hg.
- Consider treatment for blood pressures lower than this threshold if there are additional risk factors (e.g., history of cardiovascular disease, renal impairment, or previous pregnancy complications).

ACE inhibitors: (e.g., lisinopril, enalapril), angiotensin II receptor blockers (ARBs), *direct renin inhibitors* (e.g., aliskiren) should be discontinued due to risks of fetal renal damage and other adverse effects.

As per ISSHP 2021 guidelines:

- Hypertension in pregnancy should be treated with antihypertensive therapy, regardless of the underlying hypertensive disorder of pregnancy (HDP).
- Severe hypertension in pregnancy (systolic BP ≥160 mm Hg or diastolic BP ≥110 mm Hg) requires urgent antihypertensive therapy in a monitored setting.

- The target BP for antihypertensive therapy should be a diastolic BP of 85 mm Hg, irrespective of systolic BP (level of evidence: Strong).
- Nonsevere hypertension should be treated with first-line agents: Oral methyldopa, labetalol, or nifedipine (level of evidence: Strong).
- Severe hypertension should be treated with first-line agents: Oral nifedipine, oral labetalol, IV labetalol, or IV hydralazine (level of evidence: Strong).

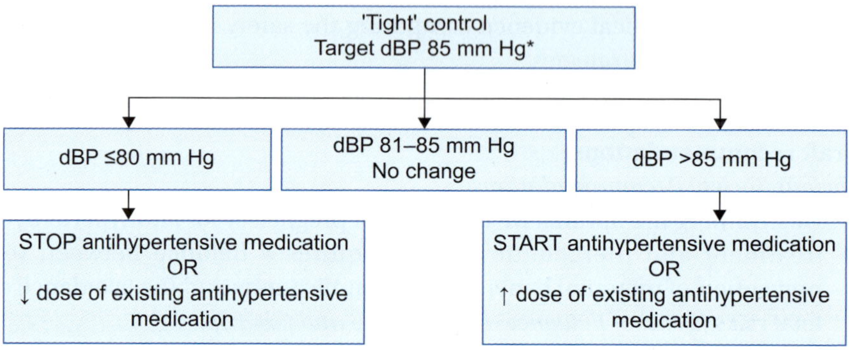

*If systolic BP (sBP) is ≥160 mm Hg, increase dose of existing medication or start new antihypertensive medication to get sBP <160 mm Hg, regardless of diastolic BP. Women require urgent treatment in a monitored setting.

Summary of evidence:

- Strict control of hypertension in pregnancy, with lower thresholds for starting antihypertensive drugs prevents and lowers the rate of preeclampsia, reduces the risk of thrombocytopenia and elevated liver enzyme levels, which are markers of disease severity. It also decreases the risk of preterm birth.
- Lowering blood pressure to below current targets (e.g., <150/90 mm Hg) in women with preeclampsia may help prevent severe neurological outcomes, such as intracerebral hemorrhage, which they may be more susceptible to, at lower systolic blood pressures compared to nonpregnant individuals.
- For pregnant women with non-severe hypertension (e.g., BPs 140–155/90–109 mm Hg) and without other severe features of preeclampsia, starting antihypertensives may allow for the prolongation of pregnancy, avoiding early delivery.
- Lowering treatment thresholds may enable timely control and reduce the need for rushed deliveries, thereby decreasing the risk of prematurity and associated complications.
- For women with preexisting conditions associated with elevated cardiovascular disease risk (e.g., diabetes, chronic kidney disease, polycystic ovary syndrome) facilitated by modern fertility techniques,

guidelines recommend more aggressive treatment due to the prevalence of chronic kidney disease and heart disease in 3% and 1% to 4% of pregnancies, respectively, in high-income countries.

- *ISSHP 2021 guidelines:* White coat hypertension (WCH) has a prevalence of 4% to 30% in pregnant individuals. Accurate diagnosis requires 24-hour ambulatory blood pressure monitoring to differentiate WCH from sustained hypertension. Women with WCH have increased risks of preeclampsia and adverse fetal outcomes compared to those with normal blood pressure, though risks are lower than those associated with sustained chronic or gestational hypertension. Regular blood pressure monitoring is essential, as nonsustained elevations can progress to sustained hypertension. Continuous follow-up is crucial and Self-measurement of blood pressure is encouraged for individuals at risk of nonsustained elevations, including WCH and masked hypertension. Early diagnosis through self-monitoring can support effective management, particularly before 20 weeks of gestation. They should have regular follow-up appointments for monitoring their blood pressure and overall health. Management strategies should be tailored to individual risk profiles.

Research gaps: Future clinical trials should address questions on the optimal BP treatment thresholds and should be adequately powered to assess the effects of different BP targets on maternal and fetal/neonatal outcomes:

- *Masked hypertension:* The frequency and impact of masked hypertension/white coat hypertension in pregnancy is not well-studied.
    - *Nonsustained BP elevations:* Any temporary increase in blood pressure during pregnancy could develop into sustained hypertension and needs monitoring.
- *International guidelines discrepancies:*
    - Variations among guidelines reflect country-specific contexts.
    - Inconsistencies hinder progress towards a global consensus on managing hypertension in pregnancy.
    - Research to define the optimal systolic and diastolic blood pressure cutoffs for initiating treatment, considering both short-term and long-term outcomes for both mother and baby.
- *Effects of home versus office BP measurements:*
    - Uncertainty about whether thresholds for starting medication based on home blood pressure measurements differ from those based on office measurements.
    - Research required to determine if self-monitoring BP thresholds should differ from office-based measurements and how these differences impact treatment decisions.

Guideline		Hypertension in pregnancy diagnosis	Treatment threshold, mm Hg	Treatment target, mm Hg	Continuation of antihypertensive therapy
ACOG	2019, 2020		≥160/105 with diagnosis of chronic hypertension ≥160/110 if acute/chronic hypertension	120–159/80–105 120–159/80–109 if chronic	Guided by informed discussion with women
World Health Organization	2018, 2020	Not defined	Not specified	Above lower limits of normal	Not specified
National Institute for Health and Care Excellence	2019		≥140/90	≤135/85	Continue treatment unless <110/70 mm Hg or symptomatic hypotension
Society of Obstetricians and Gynaecologists, Canada	2018, 2020		≥140/90	DBP, 85 <140/90+ comorbidities	Not specified
International Society for the Study of Hypertension in Pregnancy	2018	Plus, the absence of preeclampsia features	≥140/90 in office ≥135/85 at home	110–140/85	Not specified

Source:

1. Garovic VD, Dechend R, Easterling T. A Scientific Statement from the American Heart Association. Hypertension. 2022;79(2):e21-e41. Erratum in: Hypertension. 2022;79(3):e70.
2. Garcia JE, Mulrenin IR, Nguyen AB, et al. Antihypertensive medication use during pregnancy in a real-world cohort of patients diagnosed with a hypertensive disorder of pregnancy. Front Cardiovasc Med. 2023;10:1225251.

Q3. Which antihypertensives are contraindicated in pregnancy?

ACE inhibitors (e.g., lisinopril):

- *Level of evidence: High*

Angiotensin receptor blockers (ARBs) (e.g., Candesartan):

- *Level of evidence: High*

Diuretics (e.g., furosemide, hydrochlorothiazide):

- *Level of evidence: Moderate*

Beta-blocker (e.g., propranolol):

- *Level of evidence: Moderate*

Summary of evidence:

According to the Organization of Teratology Information Specialists (OTIS), the evidence regarding the use of antihypertensive drugs during pregnancy is summarized as follows:

- *ACE inhibitors:* Substantial evidence from clinical studies and case reports indicates that ACE inhibitors can cause significant fetal harm, such as urinary tract abnormalities, renal dysfunction, oligohydramnios (low amniotic fluid), and skull abnormalities. And neonatal renal failure, particularly when used in the second and third trimesters. These risks are well-documented in multiple guidelines and research studies.
- *ARBs:* They are associated with severe fetal risks including renal dysfunction, lung hypoplasia, skeletal malformations, and death. These risks are consistently reported across various studies and are widely recognized in medical guidelines.
- *Diuretics:* They can cause fetal electrolyte imbalances and may reduce placental blood flow, potentially affecting fetal growth. However, while the risks are noted, they are generally less well-studied compared to ACE inhibitors and ARBs.
- *Beta-blockers,* like propranolol, have been associated with potential risks including fetal growth restriction and bradycardia. While these risks are documented in studies, they are less severe compared to ACE inhibitors and ARBs.

Nitroprusside: Limited safety profile during pregnancy due to the risk of serious side effects, particularly fetal cyanide toxicity.

Use in practice: Last-resort medication for the urgent control of refractory severe hypertension, when other treatments have failed, and its use is usually limited to a short duration. Due to its potential risks, its administration requires close monitoring of both maternal and fetal well-being.

Research gaps:

Long-term fetal and neonatal outcomes:

- *Gap:* Limited data on the long-term effects of antihypertensive medications on child development and health.
- *Need:* More longitudinal studies to evaluate potential neurodevelopmental and cognitive impacts on children exposed to these medications in utero.

Comparative safety of different antihypertensive classes:

- *Gap:* Insufficient comparative data on the safety profiles of various antihypertensive drug classes during pregnancy.
- *Need:* Research comparing the risks and benefits of different classes of antihypertensives, such as ACE inhibitors, ARBs, beta-blockers, and others, to guide safer treatment choices.

Fetal risk assessment with newer medications:

- *Gap:* Limited research on the safety of newer antihypertensive agents and their effects on fetal development.
- *Need:* Studies to assess the safety of newer medications and their potential risks to both the fetus and the mother.

Effects of combination therapy:

- *Gap:* Insufficient evidence on the safety of using combinations of antihypertensive drugs during pregnancy.
- *Need:* Research to determine the safety and efficacy of combination therapies in managing hypertension while minimizing risks to the fetus.

Q4. What drugs are used in the management of hypertensive crisis in pregnancy?

Draft recommendations:

- *Hypertensive emergency:* Two severe BP values (≥160/110) taken 15–60 minutes apart. If severe BP elevations persist for 15 min or more, begin treatment immediately.
- Intravenous labetalol *(Level of Evidence: High)*
- Nifedipine extended release *(Level of Evidence: High)*
- Intravenous hydralazine *(Level of Evidence: Moderate)*
- Intravenous sodium nitroprusside should be reserved for refractory hypertensive emergencies in pregnancy. Hemodynamic monitoring under ICU care is required for adjusting nitroprusside administration and fluid balance. Can be considered for use when termination of pregnancy is indicated in early third trimester due to uncontrolled HTN (hypertensive crisis).

Hypertensive disorders of pregnancy (HDP)-FOGSI GCPR 2019:

- Blood pressure should be reduced to below 150 mm Hg systolic and between 80 and 100 mm Hg diastolic.
- A gradual decrease in blood pressure is advised within the first 60 minutes of treatment, targeting a systolic level of 155 to 160 mm Hg and a diastolic level of 100 to 110 mm Hg.
- IV labetalol, oral nifedipine, or IV hydralazine can be utilized to manage severe hypertension in pregnancy, as long as the healthcare provider is knowledgeable about dosing, onset of action, and potential side effects.

- Nifedipine and hydralazine may lead to tachycardia and are not recommended for patients with a heart rate exceeding 100/min; in such cases, labetalol is a better option.
- Labetalol should be avoided in patients with bradycardia (heart rate <60 bpm), asthma, or congestive heart failure; nifedipine is preferred in these scenarios.
- Magnesium sulfate not recommended as antihypertensive agent—should be used for seizure prophylaxis and controlling seizures in eclampsia.
- Nifedipine and $MgSO_4$ can be administered concurrently.
- Sublingual nifedipine is not advised.
- Diuretics are not recommended for routine use, except in specific cases such as fluid challenges in oliguria or pulmonary edema.
- In cases of severe preeclampsia, the Pritchard regimen or ZUSPAN IV regimen of $MgSO_4$ is recommended until 24 hours after delivery.
- If no IV access available, initiate oral nifedipine, or oral labetalol—200 mg and repeat in 30 min if SBP remains ≥160 or DBP ≥110 and IV access still unavailable
- *May also consider:* Labetalol or nicardipine via infusion pump
- *Sodium nitroprusside for extreme emergencies:* To be used for shortest amount of time due to cyanide/thiocyanate toxicity

Summary of evidence:

Labetalol: Used as a first-line treatment for acute management of hypertensive crises in pregnancy. It is a combined alpha- and beta-blocker with strong evidence supporting its efficacy and safety in managing severe hypertension during pregnancy. It helps in rapid blood pressure reduction and is generally well-tolerated.

Drugs used with dosages and route of administration:

- *Intravenous labetalol:*
  - *Initial dose:* 20 mg IV over 2 minutes
  - *Subsequent doses:* 40 mg IV after 10 minutes if the initial dose is not effective, followed by 80 mg every 10 minutes up to a maximum cumulative dose of 300 mg.
  - *Maintenance:* Continuous infusion at 1–2 mg/min may be considered.
- *Intravenous hydralazine:* It can cause sudden precipitous fall in blood pressure and reflex tachycardia. Hence vitals monitoring is very essential as it can also cause cardiac failure. It needs to be used in a High Dependency Unit or ICU setup where all necessary facilities and cardiac monitors are available in case of sudden complications. Infusion pump is a safe option when IV form is required for administration.
  - *Initial dose:* 5–10 mg IV over 2 minutes.
  - *Repeat doses:* 5–10 mg every 20–40 minutes if needed.
  - *Maintenance:* Continuous infusion of 0.5–10 mg/h may be used.

- *Oral nifedipine:*
  - *Immediate-release capsules:* 10 mg orally.
  - *Repeat dose:* 10–20 mg orally in 20–30 minutes if needed.
  - *Maintenance:* 10–20 mg every 4–6 hours as needed.
  - *Magnesium sulfate for seizure prophylaxis:*
  - If hypertensive crisis delivery is imminent.

Research gaps:

- Insufficient data on the long-term effects of antihypertensive drugs used during hypertensive crises on maternal and fetal health.
- Lack of consensus on optimal dosing regimens and administration routes for managing acute hypertensive crises.
- Inadequate research on how specific subpopulations (e.g., women with preexisting conditions, different ethnic groups) respond to antihypertensive treatments during crises.
  - *Need:* Targeted studies to understand how variations in patient demographics impact drug efficacy and safety.
- Variability in clinical guidelines across different regions and institutions regarding the management of hypertensive crises.
  - *Need:* Efforts to harmonize guidelines based on comprehensive, global research to provide consistent and evidence-based recommendations.
  - *ACOG Severe Hypertension 2020 Algorithm*

Labetalol Algorithm

EXAMPLE

Trigger: If severe elevations (SBP ≥160 or DBP ≥110) persist* for 15 minutes or more
OR If two severe elevations are obtained within 15 minutes and tx is clinically indicated

1. Labetalol 20 mg+ IV over 2 minutes →
2. Repeat BP In 10 minutes →
3. If SBP ≥ 160 or DBP ≥110, administer labetalol 40 mg IV over 2 minutes; If BP below threshold, continue to monitor BP closely →
4. Repeat BP In 10 minutes →
5. IF SBP ≥160 or DBP ≥110, administer labetalol 80 mg IV over 2 minutes; If BP below threshold, continue to monitor BP closely →
6. Repeat BP In 10 minutes →
7. IF SBP ≥160 or DBP ≥110, administer hydralazine§ 10 mg IV over 2 minutes; If below threshold, continue to monitor BP closely →
8. Repeat BP in 20 minutes →
9. IFSBP ≥160 or DBP ≥110 at 20 minutes, obtain emergency consultation from specialist in MFM, internal medicine, anesthesiology, or critical care →
10. Give additional antihypertensive medication per specific order as recommended by specialist →
11. Once BP thresholds are achieved, repeat BP: →
12.
    - Every 10 minutes for 1 hour
    - Then every 15 minutes for 1 hour
    - Then every 30 minutes for 1 hour
    - Then every hour for 4 hours

    → Institute additional BP monitoring per specific order

* Two severe readings more than 15 minutes and less than 60 minutes apart
\+ Avoid parenteral labetalol with active† asthma, heart disease, or congestive heart failure; use with caution with history of asthma. May cause neonatal bradycardia.
† "Active asthma" is defined as:
Ⓐ Symptoms at least once a week, or
Ⓑ Use of an inhaler, corticosteroids for asthma during the pregnancy, or
Ⓒ Any history of intubation or hospitalization for asthma.
§ Hydralazine may increase risk of maternal hypotension.

- Notify provider after one severe BP value is obtained
- Institute fetal surveillance if viable
- Hold IV labetalol for maternal pulse under 60
- Maximum cumulative IV-administered dose of labetalol should not exceed 300 mg in 24 hours
- There may be adverse effects and contraindications. Clinical judgment should prevail.

Safe Motherhood Initiative

Revised February 2020

ACOG The American College of Obstetricians and Gynecologists

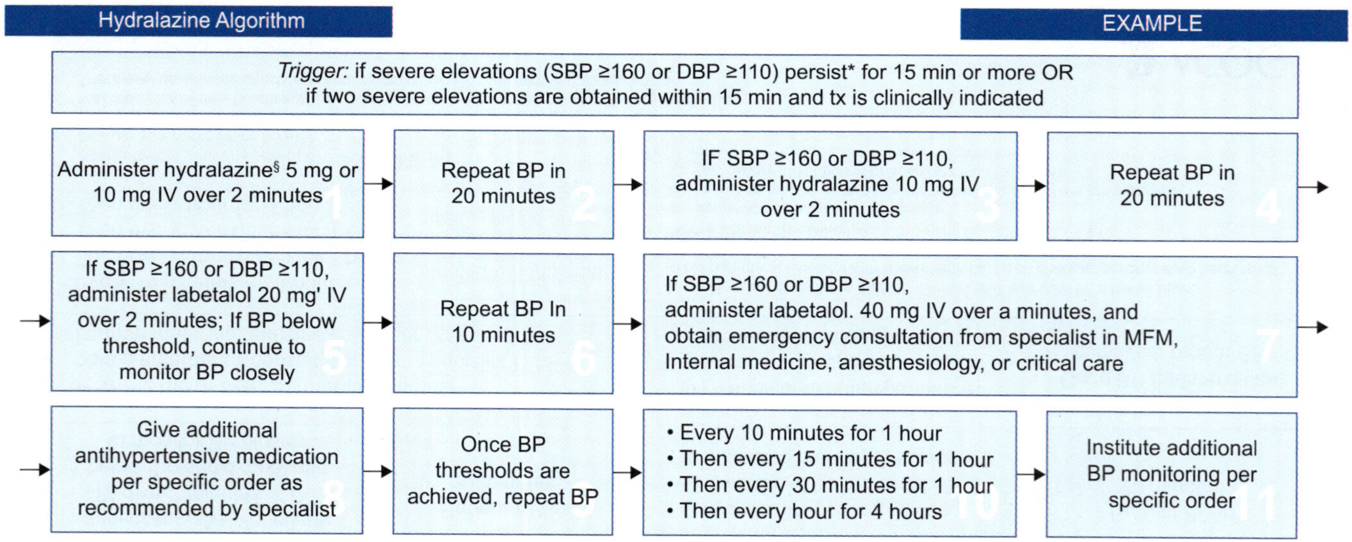

- Notify provider after one severe BP value is obtained
- Institute fetal surveillance if viable
- Hold V labetalol for maternal pulse under 60
- There may be adverse effects and contraindications.
- Clinical judgement should prevail.

* Two severe readings more than 15 minutes and less than 60 minutes apart

* Avoid parenteral labetalol with active asthma, heart disease, or congestive heart failure; use with caution with history of asthma. May cause neonatal bradycardia.

* "Active asthma" is defined as:

Ⓐ Symptoms at least once a week, or

Ⓑ Use of an inhaler, corticosteroids for asthma during the pregnancy, or

Ⓒ Any history of intubation or hospitalization for asthma.

§ Hydralazine may increase risk of maternal hypotension.

Safe Motherhood Initiative

Revised February 2020

ACOG The American College of Obstetricians and Gynecologists

Immediate-Release Oral Nifedipine Algorithm

EXAMPLE

Trigger: If severe elevations (SBP ≥160 or DBP ≥110) persist* for 15 min or more OR
If two severe elevations are obtained within 15 min and tx is clinically indicated

1. Immediate-Release Oral nifedipine§ 10 mg →
2. Repeat BP in 20 minutes →
3. If SBP ≥160 or DBP ≥ 110, administer oral nifedipine 20 mg; If below threshold, continue to monitor BP closely →
4. Repeat BP in 20 minutes →
5. If SBP ≥360 or DBP) ≥110, give additional round of oral nifedipine 20 mg →
6. Repeat BP In 20 minutes →
7. IF SBP ≥160 or DBP ≥110, administer IV labetalol 20 mg. →
8. If either BP threshold is still exceeded, administer labetalol (20 mg IV for more than 2 minutes) and obtain emergency consultation from maternal-fetal medicine, Intemal medicine, anesthesia, or critical care subspecialists. →
9. If SBP ≥160 or DBP) ≥130, give additional antihypertensive medication per specific order as recommended by specialist Obtain emergency consultation from specialist in MFM, Internal medicine, anesthesiology, or critical care. →
10. Once BP thresholds are achieved, repeat BP: →
11. • Every 10 minutes for 1 hour
    • Then every 15 minutes for 1 hour
    • Then every 30 minutes for 1 hour
    • Then every hour for 4 hours →
12. Institute additional BP monitoring per specific order

- Notify provider after one severe BP value is obtained
- Institute fetal surveillance if viable
- Capsules should be administered orally and not punctured or otherwise administered sublingually
- There may be adverse effects and contraindications. Clinical judgement should prevail.

* Two severe readings more than 15 minutes and less than 60 minutes apart

§ Immediate-release oral nifedipine has been associated with an increase in maternal heart rate and may overshoot hypertension

\+ Avoid parenteral labetalol with active asthma, heart disease, or congestive heart failure; use with caution with history of asthma. May cause neonatal bradycardia.

† "Active asthma" is defined as:

Ⓐ Symptoms at least once a week, or
Ⓑ Use of an inhaler, corticosteroids for asthma during the pregnancy, or
Ⓒ Any history of intubation or hospitalization for asthma.

Safe Motherhood Initiative

Revised February 2020

ACOG The American College of Obstetricians and Gynecologists

Q5. What are the adverse effects of antihypertensive drugs used in preeclampsia?

Draft recommendations:

1. *Labetalol (level of evidence: high):*
   Side effects:
   - *Maternal:* Dizziness, fatigue, nausea, headache, hypotension, bradycardia, and potential liver enzyme elevation.
   - *Fetal:* Possible fetal bradycardia or decreased variability in fetal heart rate.
2. *Nifedipine (level of evidence: high):*
   Side effects:
   - *Maternal:* Headache, flushing, dizziness, tachycardia, and peripheral edema.
   - *Fetal:* Rarely, transient changes in fetal heart rate may occur.
3. *Methyldopa (level of evidence: moderate):*
   Side effects:
   - *Maternal:* Sedation, dry mouth, dizziness, headache, and potential for liver dysfunction.
   - *Fetal:* Minimal direct effects, but less commonly used due to side effects and slower onset of action.

   It is less favored in current guidelines due to the availability of newer medications with better efficacy and side effect profiles. It may be considered if other agents are contraindicated.
4. *Hydralazine (level of evidence: moderate)*:
   Side effects:
   - *Maternal:* Headache, tachycardia, palpitations, nausea, hypotension, and potential for lupus-like syndrome with long-term use.
   - *Fetal:* Possible fetal tachycardia and reduced variability in fetal heart rate

Hydralazine is recommended for acute severe hypertension in preeclampsia, with careful monitoring for side effects. It is not typically used as a first-line option but can be effective when used appropriately.

5. *Aspirin (low-dose): Level of evidence: High (for prophylaxis)*:
   Side effects:
   - *Maternal:* Gastrointestinal discomfort, bleeding risks, and hypersensitivity reactions.
   - *Fetal:* Minimal risk when used at recommended doses.

Summary of evidence:

- Labetalol is recommended as a first-line antihypertensive in preeclampsia due to its proven efficacy and generally acceptable side effect profile. Regular monitoring of maternal blood pressure and fetal heart rate is advised to prevent adverse effects—
  ACOG and the Society for Maternal-Fetal Medicine (SMFM)

- Extended-release nifedipine is effective for managing moderate to severe hypertension in preeclampsia. It is recommended due to its effectiveness and lower risk of severe side effects compared to some other agents (According to ACOG and SMFM)
- Methyldopa may be used as a second-line option for hypertension management in preeclampsia. Due to its side effect profile and slower onset, it is typically not preferred for acute management but may be used in chronic cases or where other options are unsuitable.
- Hydralazine is typically reserved for acute management of severe hypertension and used in combination with other medications.
- Low-dose aspirin is recommended for the prevention of preeclampsia in high-risk pregnancies. It should be started before 16 weeks of gestation and continued until delivery (supported by ACOG and SMFM)

Research gaps:

- Insufficient research on the long-term safety of antihypertensives for the health outcomes of neonates, long term neurological development of child and health of mother, particularly for chronic use beyond pregnancy.
- Lack of research on how demographic factors (e.g., race, ethnicity, and genetic variability) influence the efficacy and safety of antihypertensives.
- Inadequate data on the effects of antihypertensives in pregnant women with comorbid conditions such as diabetes, autoimmune disorders, or chronic kidney disease.
- Lack of comprehensive studies on newer or alternative antihypertensive medications and their safety profiles in pregnancy.

8.2 ANTICONVULSANTS

Vidya Thobbi

Q1. What is the role of anticonvulsant drugs in preeclampsia?

Draft recommendations:

Seizure prophylaxis:

- Magnesium sulfate is the first-line treatment for the prevention of seizures in women with severe preeclampsia and is the first line treatment for eclamptic seizures
- It should be initiated in all women diagnosed with severe preeclampsia, defined by criteria such as systolic blood pressure ≥160 mm Hg or diastolic blood pressure ≥110 mm Hg, along with evidence of end-organ dysfunction or fetal distress.
- Magnesium treatment should be continued for at least 24 hours after a patient's last convulsion or delivery whichever is later—*FOGSI GCPR*
- Other antiepileptic medications include diazepam or phenytoin.

- Benzodiazepines and barbiturates are used for refractory seizures that are unresponsive to magnesium.
- Levetiracetam or valproic acid are alternatives for patients with myasthenia gravis with eclampsia as magnesium and phenytoin cause increased muscle weakness, which could lead to a myasthenia crisis.

Postpartum management:

- Approximately a third of eclamptic seizures occur postpartum, seizure prophylaxis with magnesium sulfate or alternate anticonvulsant should be continued for at least 24 hours after delivery.
- Inpatient observation or close home monitoring is recommended for 72 hours postpartum.
- *Treatment threshold*:
    - Systolic BP of 150 mm Hg or greater. Diastolic BP of 100 mm Hg or greater.
    - Measurements should be taken on two occasions at least four hours apart.
    - If systolic BP is 160 mm Hg or greater or diastolic BP is 110 mm Hg or greater, recheck within 15 minutes.
    - Initiate treatment within 60 minutes if BP remains elevated after the recheck.
    - *Common medications used*: Oral nifedipine or labetalol, intravenous labetalol or hydralazine
    - The ACOG suggests that women with gestational hypertension or preeclampsia receive BP monitoring up to 72 hours postpartum and again 7 to 10 days after delivery, or sooner with symptoms. Preeclampsia and eclampsia can occur up to 4 weeks postpartum, all women should be educated on warning signs and evaluated promptly for potential hypertensive complications.

Patient and family education: Educate patients and their families about the signs of potential complications associated with magnesium sulfate therapy and the importance of reporting any unusual symptoms promptly.

Multidisciplinary approach: Ensure comprehensive management of severe preeclampsia by using a collaborative approach involving obstetricians, maternal-fetal medicine specialists, and neonatologists.

Summary of evidence: Eclampsia is defined as the new onset of generalized tonic-clonic seizures in a woman with preeclampsia. Eclamptic seizures can occur antepartum, 20 weeks after gestation, intrapartum, and postpartum. Seizures before 20 weeks are rare but have been documented in gestational trophoblastic disease.

A significant body of evidence attests to the efficacy of magnesium sulfate to prevent seizures in women with preeclampsia with severe features and eclampsia. In the Magpie study, a randomized placebo-controlled trial with 10,110 participants (two thirds originating from developing countries), the seizure rate was reduced overall by more than one half with this treatment.

Magnesium sulfate ($MgSO_4$) is widely recognized as the *gold standard* for managing eclampsia.

Effectiveness: Research indicates that $MgSO_4$ is superior to other medications in controlling seizures associated with eclampsia, significantly lowering the incidence of recurrent seizures, eclamptic fatalities, and associated complications.

Administration: The administration of $MgSO_4$ can be performed by trained healthcare personnel who are also capable of monitoring for potential side effects, ensuring patient safety.

Mechanism: $MgSO_4$ acts by limiting the formation of edema through the restriction of water and solute movement into the brain. Additionally, it reduces pinocytosis, which is heightened during episodes of acute hypertension.

Magnesium sulfate effectiveness: It is more effective than phenytoin, diazepam, or nimodipine in preventing eclampsia.

Preferred drug: Magnesium sulfate should be the first choice for preventing eclampsia antepartum and after delivery.

Alternative medications:

- *Benzodiazepines and phenytoin:*
  - These should only be used if magnesium sulfate is contraindicated or not available.
  - They are primarily considered for antiepileptic treatment.

Contraindications for magnesium sulfate:

- Do not use magnesium sulfate in the following conditions:
  - Myasthenia gravis
  - Hypocalcemia
  - Moderate-to-severe renal failure
  - Cardiac ischemia
  - Heart block
  - Myocarditis

Q2. What are the different regimes used for anticonvulsant drugs in preeclampsia?

Draft recommendations:

- Magnesium sulfate remains the drug of choice for both prevention and treatment of women with eclampsia. (*Level of Evidence: A*—Based on multiple randomized controlled trials and meta-analyses showing efficacy in reducing seizure recurrence and improving maternal and neonatal outcomes.)

- Do not use diazepam, phenytoin or other anticonvulsants as an alternative to magnesium sulfate in women with eclampsia (*Level of Evidence: C*)
- The Zuspan regimen is generally safe when administered with appropriate monitoring.
  - *Level of Evidence: A* (Evidence from clinical studies and guidelines supports the safety of the Zuspan regimen, provided that monitoring for magnesium toxicity is strictly adhered to)
- The Pritchard regimen is a protocol for administering magnesium sulfate ($MgSO_4$) to manage severe preeclampsia and is designed to be practical, particularly in settings where intravenous administration may not be feasible.

Summary of evidence: *NICE/RCOG guidelines*: Use the Collaborative Eclampsia Trial regimen for administration of magnesium sulfate:

A loading dose of 4 g should be given intravenously over 5 to 15 minutes, followed by an infusion of 1 g/hour maintained for 24 hours. If the woman has had an eclamptic fit, the infusion should be continued for 24 hours after the last fit.

Recurrent fits should be treated with a further dose of 2 g to 4 g given intravenously over 5 to 15 minutes.

The Zuspan regimen: The Zuspan regimen is a well-supported protocol for magnesium sulfate administration in eclampsia, with proven efficacy and safety when administered with careful monitoring. It is a viable option among different magnesium sulfate regimens, and its use should be tailored to patient needs and institutional guidelines.

The regimen has a favorable safety profile when compared to other protocols, assuming proper monitoring is in place. Magnesium toxicity, though manageable, is a potential risk, but careful adherence to dosing and monitoring protocols minimizes this risk.

- *Loading dose:* Administer 4 grams of magnesium sulfate intravenously over 15–20 minutes.
- *Maintenance dose:* Following the loading dose, administer a continuous intravenous infusion of magnesium sulfate at a rate of 1 gram per hour.

Other regimens:

- *Pritchard regimen*
- *Loading dose:* Administer 4 grams of magnesium sulfate intravenously over 5-10 minutes.
- Additionally, give 10 grams of magnesium sulfate intramuscularly, with 5 g in each buttock.

- *Maintenance dose:* Administer 5 g of magnesium sulfate intramuscularly every 4 hours in alternate buttocks.
- *Duration:* Continue the magnesium sulfate regimen for 24 hours after delivery or the last seizure, whichever is later.

NICE/RCOG guidelines: Green Top Guideline No 68:
Sibai's regimen:

1. *Loading dose:* A common initial dose is 4–6 grams of magnesium sulfate administered intravenously over 15–30 minutes.
2. *Maintenance dose:* After the loading dose, a continuous infusion of 1–2 grams per hour is usually administered.
3. *Duration:* Treatment is typically continued for 24 hours after delivery or the last seizure if used for eclampsia.

The *Dhaka regimen* is a simplified protocol for administering magnesium sulfate ($MgSO_4$) for the management of severe pre-eclampsia and eclampsia. It is designed to be more feasible for use in low-resource settings. The regimen includes both intramuscular and intravenous routes and is as follows (RCOG Green-top Guideline No. 46)

1. *Loading dose:* 14 grams of $MgSO_4$, administered intravenously (IV) or intramuscularly (IM) over 20 minutes.
2. *Maintenance dose:* 5 grams IM every 6 hours for up to 24 hours after the last seizure.

Use of *other anticonvulsants* such as valproic acid or benzodiazepines is not generally recommended for routine management of eclampsia.

- *Level of Evidence: C*—Based on limited evidence and expert consensus, indicating that these agents are not typically preferred due to lack of robust evidence supporting their efficacy and safety in this specific context. They may be considered in exceptional circumstances or as adjuncts if specific clinical scenarios arise.
- Diazepam was introduced for treatment of eclampsia based on the belief that a traditional anticonvulsant would be the effective. Diazepam binds to a specific site of the γ-aminobutyric $acid_A$ ($GABA_A$) receptor, the major inhibitory neurotransmitter in the central nervous system. The $GABA_A$ receptor is an inhibitory channel which, when activated, decreases neuronal activity. The anticonvulsant properties of diazepam may be in part or entirely due to binding to voltage-dependent sodium channels. Diazepam has near immediate onset of action, as it rapidly crosses the blood brain barrier, with a short duration of action (20 to 30 minutes) and half-life time of elimination of 20 to 50 hours. Drug elimination is prolonged in neonates, the elderly and those with liver dysfunction.
- Diazepam is primarily eliminated by liver enzymes, hence its many potential drug interactions. While short-term use of diazepam is

generally well tolerated, common side effects are drowsiness, confusion and amnesia.

- Treatment with diazepam usually includes a loading dose of 40 mg by intravenous injection, followed by an infusion of 20 mg diluted in 500 mL. This infusion is titrated against the level of sedation, with the aim of keeping the woman drowsy but rousable.
- Women allocated magnesium sulfate had a 52% lower risk of recurrent convulsions (95% Cl 64% to 37% reduction) than those allocated diazepam (60 [13·2%] vs. 126 [27·9%]; i.e., 14·7 [SD 2·6] fewer women with recurrent convulsions per 100 women; 2p<0·00001).
- Women allocated magnesium sulfate were also less likely to be ventilated, to develop pneumonia, and to be admitted to intensive care facilities than those allocated phenytoin. The babies of women who had been allocated magnesium sulfate before delivery were significantly less likely to be intubated at the place of delivery, and to be admitted to a special care nursery, than the babies of mothers who had been allocated phenytoin according to studies.
- *Levetiracetam* is a newer anticonvulsant. It has been used extensively in pregnancy as an anticonvulsant drug in epileptic women. It has been proven to be safe in pregnancy and has shown not to have any adverse effects on the fetus. Levetiracetam has a 12 hourly dosage and does not need extensive monitoring as in comparison to magnesium sulfate. It has been used as a second-line anticonvulsant in eclampsia.
- Levetiracetam is an antiepileptic drug that works through various mechanisms such as inhibition of voltage-dependent N-type calcium channels, binding to synaptic proteins that modulate neurotransmitter release and facilitation of GABAergic inhibition.
- A retrospective study conducted in the US showed that levetiracetam was being used in the prevention of convulsions in preeclampsia more so in those patients who had contraindications to the administration of magnesium sulfate like rising serum creatine and serum magnesium sulfate, pulmonary edema, reduced urine output or symptoms like headache, vision changes. In another retrospective study conducted in Mumbai, India, it was seen that levetiracetam was administered in eclamptic patients who had low urine output or who had convulsions after the administration of magnesium sulfate. They have shown favorable results with levetiracetam. Levetiracetam has been mentioned as a drug that can be used in eclampsia where magnesium sulfate is contraindicated. Levetiracetam may be of great use in remote places where monitoring of the adverse effects of magnesium sulfate may not be possible. It may be of great importance in those patients who already have clinical features that are contraindicated for the administration of magnesium sulfate.

- As it is a pilot study, larger studies are required in his field.
- *Lamotrigine:* While some studies suggest that lamotrigine can be effective in controlling seizures, most research supports magnesium sulfate as the first-line treatment due to its well-documented efficacy in preventing eclamptic seizures.
- A few case reports and small studies indicate that lamotrigine may be beneficial, particularly in women with a history of epilepsy or those who are unable to tolerate magnesium sulfate. The contraindications and potential risks associated with its use necessitate careful consideration and monitoring. Continued research is essential to better understand its role compared to magnesium sulfate.

Q3. What are the side effects of anticonvulsant drugs?

Draft recommendations:

Serum magnesium levels should remain within a range of 0.7 to 1 mmol/L (1.4 to 2.0 mEq/L) concentration, but almost half of the total body magnesium is taken up by the bone.

Hypermagnesemia is a state of elevated magnesium levels with serum concentrations higher than 2 mmol/L.

1. *Magnesium sulfate ($MgSO_4$):*

   Common side effects:
   - *Flushing:* Warmth and redness of the skin.
   - *Nausea and vomiting:* Common gastrointestinal symptoms.
   - *Headache:* Often due to vasodilation

   Serious side effects:
   - *Magnesium toxicity:* Symptoms include loss of deep tendon reflexes, respiratory depression, hypotension, and altered mental status.
   - *Respiratory depression*
   - *Cardiovascular effects:* Bradycardia and hypotension

   Management: Regular monitoring of serum magnesium levels, vital signs, and clinical symptoms is essential to avoid toxicity. Treatment includes discontinuation of $MgSO_4$ and administration of calcium gluconate or calcium chloride as an antidote.
2. *Phenytoin*:

   Common side effects:
   - *Gingival hyperplasia:* Overgrowth of gum tissue.
   - *Rash:* Skin rashes can develop.
   - *Drowsiness and ataxia:* Sedation and coordination problems

   Serious side effects:
   - *Stevens-Johnson syndrome:* A severe, potentially life-threatening skin reaction.

- *Hepatotoxicity:* Liver damage can occur, particularly with prolonged use.
- *Hypotension:* Can result from rapid intravenous administration.

Management: Regular monitoring of liver function and blood levels. Avoid rapid IV infusion and monitor for signs of severe skin reactions.

3. *Other anticonvulsants (if used as adjunctive therapy)*:
   Common side effects:
   - *Sedation:* Drowsiness and fatigue.
   - *Gastrointestinal disturbances:* Nausea, vomiting, and abdominal pain.

   Serious side effects:
   - *Rash:* Risk of serious skin reactions like Stevens-Johnson syndrome.
   - *Hematologic issues:* Changes in blood cell counts.

Summary of evidence: Magnesium levels must be monitored clinically by checking patellar reflexes or urinary output.

- *Normal serum levels:* 0.7–1.0 mmol/L (1.4–2.0 mEq/L)
- *Therapeutic level in preeclampsia/eclampsia:* 2.0–3.5 mmol/L (4–7 mEq/L)
- *Patellar reflexes lost:* 4.0–5.0 mmol/L (8–10 mEq/L)
- *Respiratory paralysis:* 6.0–7.5 mmol/L (12–15 mEq/L)
- *Cardiac arrest:* 12.5–15.0 mmol/L (25–30 mEq/L)

Minor side effects seen early on in hypermagnesemia include flushed skin, nausea or vomiting, and generalized muscle weakness.

As magnesium levels increase, the muscle weakness progresses to loss of deep tendon reflexes and, eventually, flaccid paralysis that can cause respiratory compromise.

Further complications include those in the cardiovascular system, beginning with hypotension and bradycardia. If magnesium levels remain uncorrected, this can lead to a complete heart block and, subsequently, cardiac arrest.

Magnesium sulfate is the primary anticonvulsant used in managing eclampsia.

Although other medications are not typically first-line treatments for seizures, they may be used in specific cases or as adjuncts.

Each of these medications has its own side effect profile, necessitating careful management. Effective monitoring and adherence to dosing guidelines are essential for minimizing and managing these potential side effects.

Q4. What is magnesium toxicity and its management?

Draft recommendations:

- Adhere to established dosing regimens, such as the Prichard or Zuspan protocols, to minimize the risk of magnesium toxicity.

- Frequently check vital signs, and clinical status to ensure that magnesium concentrations remain within the limits.
- Watch for early signs of magnesium toxicity, including loss of deep tendon reflexes, respiratory depression, hypotension, and changes in mental status.
- Immediately Cease Magnesium Sulfate Infusion if toxicity is suspected.
- Provide calcium gluconate (1 g IV over 2–5 minutes) or calcium chloride (1 g IV over 2–5 minutes) as an antidote to counteract magnesium toxicity. Supportive care, including oxygen therapy, may also be necessary.
- Maintain monitoring of serum magnesium levels, vital signs, and clinical status following antidote administration to ensure recovery and prevent recurrence of toxicity.
- Evaluate renal function, as impaired renal function can affect magnesium metabolism and clearance, increasing the risk of toxicity.

Summary of evidence: High levels of magnesium in the blood can be toxic and cause serious symptoms that worsen as levels increase:

- *5–10 mEq/L:* ECG changes such as a prolonged PR interval and widened QRS complex start to appear.
- *10 mEq/L:* Loss of deep tendon reflexes and muscle weakness occur.
- *15 mEq/L:* Abnormal heart rhythms, including SA/AV node block, may develop, and respiratory paralysis can happen.
- *20 mEq/L or higher:* The risk of cardiac arrest becomes high.

The severity of symptoms is directly related to the concentration of magnesium in the blood.

Serum magnesium level: A serum magnesium level greater than *7.0 mg/dL (1.5 mmol/L)* indicates a risk of toxicity. Most guidelines recommend stopping the infusion if levels exceed this threshold.

Clinical signs of toxicity:

- *Respiratory depression:* Respiratory rate less than 12 breaths per minute or significant decrease in respiratory effort.
- *Hypotension:* Blood pressure that drops significantly or becomes unstable.
- *Loss of deep tendon reflexes:* The absence of reflexes, particularly the patellar reflex, indicates significant magnesium accumulation.
- *Altered mental status:* Confusion, lethargy, or decreased level of consciousness.
- *Cardiac arrhythmias:* Any arrhythmias observed on an ECG.

Neuromuscular symptoms:

- *Loss of deep tendon reflexes:* This is often one of the earliest signs of toxicity. In obese patients where there may be difficulty in eliciting knee jerk, below mentioned are the other alternative clinical ways to elicit deep tendon reflexes before attributing it to $MgSO_4$ toxicity.

Biceps reflex:
Description: Tapping the biceps tendon at the elbow assesses the C5-C6 nerve roots

Triceps reflex:
Description: Tapping the triceps tendon at the elbow evaluates the C6-C7 nerve roots

Ankle jerk reflex (Achilles reflex):
Description: This reflex can be assessed by tapping the Achilles tendon, though it may also be challenging in obese patients.

Plantar reflex:
Description: Stroking the sole of the foot to observe for the Babinski response or normal toe flexion.

Supinator (brachioradialis) reflex:
Description: Tapping the brachioradialis tendon near the wrist assesses the C5-C6 nerve roots.

Abdominal reflex:
- *Description*: Gently stroking the skin of the abdomen to elicit contraction of the abdominal muscles
- Muscle weakness
- Respiratory depression
- *Flaccid paralysis:* In severe cases, paralysis may occur.

Cardiovascular symptoms:
- Hypotension
- Bradycardia
- Cardiac arrhythmias
- Cardiac arrest

Central nervous system symptoms:
- Confusion
- Lethargy
- *Coma:* In severe cases

Other symptoms:
- *Nausea and vomiting:* These can occur due to gastrointestinal irritation.
- Flushing
- Oliguria or anuria—can be indicative of kidney dysfunction.

The antidote for magnesium sulfate toxicity is calcium gluconate. It is administered intravenously to counteract the effects of magnesium toxicity.

Dosage and administration:
Calcium gluconate dose: The typical dose is 1 gram (10 mL of a 10% solution) administered intravenously over 2–5 minutes. The exact dose and rate of

administration may depend on the severity of the toxicity and the clinical scenario.

Research gaps: Current guidelines for anticonvulsants offer general dosing recommendations, but there is significant variability in practice, with limited research on optimal dosing and administration protocols. The safety and effectiveness of anticonvulsants, especially magnesium sulfate ($MgSO_4$), in special populations—such as those with co-existing conditions like renal or cardiac issues—are not well understood. There is no established clinically effective magnesium concentration for preventing eclampsia, and the optimal dosing regimen for magnesium sulfate has not been determined due to a lack of standard pharmacological studies.

Long-term maternal and neonatal outcomes with magnesium sulfate use for eclampsia are under-researched, and while short-term adverse effects are known, the long-term impacts on maternal health and the neonate require further study. Additionally, there is limited research on how genetic factors and comorbidities influence the safety and efficacy of $MgSO_4$, as well as the potential interactions between magnesium sulfate and other medications used in eclampsia, such as antihypertensives.

There is also a need for more standardized protocols for monitoring magnesium sulfate levels, clinical signs of toxicity, and for managing and reversing toxicity. Research into alternative anticonvulsants is limited, particularly for cases where magnesium sulfate is contraindicated or ineffective. Overall, more research is needed to refine dosing protocols, understand individual variability in response, and improve management strategies for magnesium sulfate in the treatment of eclampsia.

BIBLIOGRAPHY

1. ACOG. Practice Bulletin No. 207: Eclampsia. Obstet Gynecol. 2020;135(5):e166-76.
2. American College of Obstetricians and Gynaecologists. Hypertension in pregnancy. Report of the American College of Obstetricians and Gynecologists' Task Force on Hypertension in Pregnancy. Obstet Gynecol. 2013;122(5):1122-31.
3. Khalil A, Bhandari A, Lee A, et al. Levetiracetam for the treatment of seizures in pregnancy: a systematic review. Eur J Obstet Gynecol Reprod Biol. 2019;240:204-9.
4. Kirkpatrick D, et al. Mechanisms of magnesium sulfate neuroprotection in preeclampsia and eclampsia. Am J Obstet Gynecol. 2016;214(4):470.e1-470.e10.
5. Markham K, Funai EF. Pregnancy-related hypertension. In: Creasy RK, Resnik R, Iams JD (Eds). Creasy and Resnik's Maternal-Fetal Medicine, 7th edition. Philadelphia: Elsevier; 2015. pp. 756-81.
6. Prasannan L, Blitz MJ, Rochelson BL, et al. Contraindications to magnesium sulfate and alternative seizure prophylaxis for severe preeclampsia [09L]. Obstet Gynecol. 2020;135:126S.

7. Satia M, Shilotri M. A study of the obstetric and perinatal outcomes of eclampsia and the use of levetiracetam in its management. Int J Reprod Contracept Obstet Gynecol. 2016;5(12):4266-70.
8. Sutton ALM, Harper LM, Tita ATN. Hypertensive Disorders in Pregnancy. Obstet Gynecol Clin North Am. 2018;45(2):333-47.
9. Waters J. Management of Myasthenia Gravis in Pregnancy. Neurol Clin. 2019;37(1):113-20.
10. Which anticonvulsant for women with eclampsia? Evidence from the Collaborative Eclampsia Trial. Lancet. 1995;345(8963):1455-63.

CHAPTER 9

Decision to Deliver in Hypertensive Disorders in Pregnancy

Suchitra Pandit

INTRODUCTION

Hypertensive disorders of pregnancy (HDP) are a leading cause of maternal and fetal morbidity and mortality worldwide. These disorders complicate up to 10% of pregnancies and are a significant contributor to preterm birth, low birth weight, and maternal mortality.

Standard management of preeclampsia involves maternal and fetal assessment and subsequent consideration of timely delivery to minimize maternal and perinatal morbidity, taking into consideration gestational age, progression of maternal disease, and fetal well-being.

The decision to deliver should involve balancing the risks of worsening preeclampsia against those of prematurity. The potential benefits and risks should be discussed with the mother as part of a shared decision-making process. It will also depend on the stage of pregnancy and the health of the mother and baby.

KEY QUESTIONS

When to deliver:

Timely delivery based on gestational age, severity, and availability of a well-equipped hospital with a neonatal intensive care unit is important so if facilities are lacking, an in utero transfer to a tertiary care unit is recommended. The timing, place of delivery, and method of delivery influence the outcome of both the mother and the baby.

Q1. When should delivery occur?

The decision to deliver should be carefully decided after assessing maternal and fetal risks.

Preeclampsia:

Nonsevere preeclampsia (mild-to-moderate preeclampsia): Pregnancy can be continued till term with vigilant monitoring and allow spontaneous labor or induction after 37 completed weeks. Most guidelines recommend delivery after 37 weeks, because maternal risks can be reduced without additional perinatal risks

Deliver patient at or before 37 weeks, if:

- Fetal growth restriction
- Severe oligoamnios
- Maternal complications like sudden rise of high blood pressure, imminent eclampsia, or any signs suggesting severity of condition

Deliver after 37 weeks (may occur spontaneously or may be induced):

- Stable and well-controlled blood pressure
- No fetal growth restriction
- No maternal complications

In case of severe preeclampsia:
Deliver before 34 weeks if maternal conditions like:

- Severe persistent hypertension (>160/110 mm Hg) despite medication
- HELLP syndrome
- Eclampsia
- Maternal complications (e.g., stroke, cardiac failure)
- Abruptio placentae
- Severe oligoamnios

And/or
Fetal conditions like: Fetal growth restriction or abnormal Doppler suggestive of reversed end diastolic flow.

If period of gestation is between 34 and 37 weeks: Definitive treatment of preeclampsia is the delivery of the fetus. But in women with late preterm preeclampsia (between 34 and 37 weeks' gestation), the optimal time for delivery is less clear, as delivery is the appropriate treatment for severe preeclampsia, but not for the preterm fetus. So expectant management can be offered.

Current usual practice in the UK for women with late preterm preeclampsia is for expectant management until 37 weeks' gestation, with delivery sooner if the clinical scenario changes and there is concern over impending severe preeclampsia and associated complications.

Q2. What is expectant management?

Expectant management is a conservative approach to treating preeclampsia that involves delaying labor induction and taking certain medications to reduce the risk of neonatal death and morbidity. It is commonly used for preterm preeclampsia to help in achieving more fetal maturity. One has to balance the risks of maternal disease progression against complications for the neonate either related to ongoing expectant management or those related to planned earlier delivery (neonatal immaturity and associated complications).

Neonatal and maternal outcomes may benefit from delivery or expectant management, provided it is carried out in a well-equipped center with strict monitoring of the mother and fetus. Informed decision-making regarding benefits and risks of expectant management must be discussed with the patient.

Findings that indicate expeditious delivery after stabilization, regardless of gestational age, can be described as fetal and maternal factors.

Q3. How is monitoring done during expectant management?

Patient is admitted and close monitoring of maternal and fetal conditions is done with a low threshold for delivery if maternal or fetal deterioration is suspected.

This involves vigilant monitoring of vital symptoms, blood pressure, respiratory rate and urine output.

- Weekly laboratory values (CBC, platelet counts, urine for protein, liver function tests, serum creatinine, coagulation profile if thrombocytopenia, LDH, SFlt/PlGF ratio)
- Serial ultrasonography
- Deliver at 37 weeks

Q4. What are the indications for expediting delivery during expectant management?

During expectant management, delivery is recommended at any time in the case of deterioration of maternal or fetal condition, *irrespective of gestational age after maternal stabilization.*

Following criteria are to be considered:
Maternal:

- Uncontrolled severe-range blood pressure (persistent systolic BP 160 mm Hg or more or diastolic BP 110 mm Hg or more not responsive to antihypertensive medication)
- Persistent headaches, refractory to treatment
- Inability to control maternal blood pressure despite using 3 or more classes of antihypertensives in appropriate doses
- Epigastric pain or right upper pain unresponsive to repeat analgesics
- Visual disturbances, motor deficit, or altered sensorium
- Stroke
- Myocardial infarction
- HELLP syndrome
- New or worsening renal dysfunction (serum creatinine greater than 1.1 mg/dL or twice baseline)
- Pulmonary edema
- Eclampsia

- Maternal pulse oximetry less than 90%
- Suspected acute placental abruption or vaginal bleeding in the absence of placenta previa

Fetal:

- Severe fetal growth restriction
- Persistent reversed end-diastolic flow in the umbilical artery
- Fetal death
- Fetus without expectation for survival at the time of maternal diagnosis (e.g., lethal anomaly, extreme prematurity)

Q5. What is the mode of management if severe preeclampsia sets in before 25 weeks' gestation?

- If preeclampsia sets in before 25 weeks of gestation it is advisable to stabilize the patient and deliver her.
- The delivery is associated with minimal short-term maternal morbidities, although neonatal morbidity and death are high, so induction of labor is considered if the cervix is favorable especially in cases of severe preeclampsia.
- If a patient is having eclampsia, she should be stabilized after $MgSO_4$ and antihypertensives and then delivered.
- If she is already in labor, a forewater amniotomy can be done and labor can be augmented with oxytocin.
- Investigate cause of hypertension before discharging the patient.

Q6. When should a pregnant woman with chronic hypertension (HTN) be delivered?

- If a pregnant woman having chronic hypertension is well controlled on the antihypertensive drugs and the fetal growth is satisfactory, there is no need to offer delivery before 37 weeks unless there is superimposed preeclampsia or any other medical indications.
- In such women, timing of birth should be decided after discussion with her. A spontaneous labor can be awaited up to 38 weeks.
- If planned early birth is necessary offer a course of antenatal corticosteroids if before 34 weeks of gestation to enhance lung maturity.
- If between 26 and 32 weeks, offer steroids and magnesium sulfate for neuroprotection.
- The recommended time to deliver a woman with chronic hypertension depends on the stability of her condition, medications that she is using, whether she required frequent medication adjustments and if there is superimposed preeclampsia:
- Delivery timing should weigh maternal and neonatal outcomes in each gestational week with the recognition that many factors likely influence

optimal delivery timing; however, in a stable patient with mild chronic hypertension, delivery at 39 weeks of gestation may optimize outcomes.

Women with isolated chronic hypertension, induction of labor at 38 or 39 weeks of gestation may prevent complications of severe hypertensive without increasing the risk of cesarean delivery.

Q7. How will you decide about the timing of delivery?

- In case of chronic hypertension which is well controlled on antihypertensive medications, delivery less than 37 weeks is not recommended
- If there is chronic HTN with superimposed preeclampsia without severe features
  - Expectant management with delivery at 37 weeks can be offered
- If there is chronic HTN with superimposed preeclampsia with severe features:
  - Expectant management under certain circumstances until delivery at 34 weeks (inpatient care only)
  - Initiation of antenatal steroids as per guidelines

  Expectant management beyond 39 weeks of gestation should only be done after careful consideration of the risks and benefits and with appropriate surveillance.

Q8. How should such women be delivered?

Mode of delivery depends upon the urgency to deliver, cervical Bishop's score, gestational age, severity of fetal growth restriction, and Doppler study findings in the umbilical artery.

Spontaneous onset of labor (SOL) versus induction of labor (IOL):
Allow SOL:

- Nonsevere preeclampsia
- Stable blood pressure
- Fetal monitoring normal
- Gestational age ≥ 37 weeks

Induction of labor: Induction of labor should be offered to mothers eligible for vaginal delivery. Prostaglandins (PGs) (dinoprostone gel, suppositories, or tablets) can be used for induction. Misoprostol may be used in patients remote from term. Mechanical dilatation of the cervix with Foley's balloon or vaginal hygroscopic dilators may be considered. Augmentation of labor is to be done only with oxytocin.

Recommend IOL:

- Severe preeclampsia
- Fetal growth restriction
- Abnormal fetal monitoring

- Maternal complications
- Gestational age ≥34 weeks (severe) or ≥37 weeks (non-severe)

Q9. What would be indications for a cesarean delivery?

Cesarean section is done for:

- Any obstetric indication
- Failed induction
- Previous uterine surgery
- Fetal distress
- Severe FGR or reversed end-diastolic flow in the umbilical artery on color Doppler
- Severe preeclampsia with complications

Q10. How to monitor after delivery?

Risk to the mother persists after the delivery and hence monitoring is to be emphasized even after delivery:

- Continue antihypertensive treatment if required
- Antihypertensive treatment must be altered if their blood pressure falls below 130/80 mm Hg
- If a woman has taken labetalol/nifedipine to treat gestational hypertension, it must be stopped within 2 days after the birth and changed to an alternative treatment if necessary
- Use of an angiotensin-converting enzyme (ACE) inhibitor as first-line treatment is recommended.
- The choice of a second-line medicine would be beta-blockers. Angiotensin receptor blockers, thiazide, and thiazide-like diuretics are not recommended during breastfeeding.
- The medicines with once-daily administration should be used wherever enalapril in preference to captopril (which is taken 3 times daily) and atenolol as an alternative to labetalol (which is taken 2 to 4 times daily).
- For women with gestational hypertension who did not take antihypertensive treatment and have given birth, start antihypertensive treatment if their blood pressure is 150/100 mm Hg or higher.
- Offer all women who have had gestational hypertension a medical review with their specialist 6–8 weeks after the birth.
- If hypertension is related to the kidney, appropriate referral to the nephrologist.
- Lifestyle changes, weight reduction if body mass index is high. Contraception discussed and preconceptual counseling recommended if future pregnancy desired.

BIBLIOGRAPHY

1. American College of Obstetricians and Gynecologists. Gestational Hypertension and Preeclampsia: ACOG Practice Bulletin: Number 222. Obstet Gynecol. 2020;135:e237-60.
2. Bernardes TP, Zwertbroek EF, Broekhuijsen K. Delivery or expectant management for prevention of adverse maternal and neonatal outcomes in hypertensive disorders of pregnancy: an individual participant data meta-analysis. Ultrasound Obstet Gynecol. 2019;53:443-53.
3. Chappell LC, Brocklehurst P, Green ME, et al. Planned early delivery or expectant management for late preterm pre-eclampsia (PHOENIX): a randomised controlled trial. Lancet. 2019;394:1181-90.
4. NICE Guidelines NG 133. (2019). Guidelines on delivery, planning, including the use of Caesarean section.
5. The International Society for the Study of Hypertension in Pregnancy. The hypertensive disorders of pregnancy: ISSHP classification, diagnosis and management recommendations for international practice. Pregnancy Hypertens. 2021.

CHAPTER 10

Intrapartum Care in Preeclampsia

Mitra Saxena

INTRODUCTION

A preeclampsia patient is at high risk of developing life-threatening complications both for mother and baby during course of labor, so deserves continuous monitoring for maternal and fetal well-being with timely safe delivery.

Patient education about the onset of labor, pain relief, place of delivery, monitoring of mother and baby, and respectful maternity care needs to be followed diligently.

The NICE guidelines 2023, Hypertension in pregnancy: diagnosis and management published in 2019 and updated in 2023, NICE guidelines on Intrapartum Care 2023, ACOG Practice Bulletin 222, FOGSI-GESTOSIS-ICOG Hypertensive Disorders in Pregnancy (HDP) Good Clinical Practice Recommendations 2019, and Operational Guidelines for Obstetric ICUs and HDUs 2017 were reviewed to arrive at draft recommendations for the key questions to propose evidence-based *intrapartum care in preeclampsia.*

Q1. What is the required level of setup to deliver a patient of preeclampsia?

In view of the fact that preeclampsia is a high risk pregnancy with potential for adverse maternal and or fetal outcome , birth has to be planned in a well-equipped obstetric unit, with continuous monitoring for mother and baby and availability of facilities for neonatal intensive care unit, anesthesia, access to laboratory services, blood components and easy referrals to high dependency/critical care unit in case required.

Q2. What should be the components of labor room preparedness?

It is recommended that the obstetric unit be equipped with necessary equipment, medications, and personnel.

Well-calibrated equipment for blood pressure monitoring, pulse oximeter, fetal Doppler, cardiotocograph, suction, oxygen, medications for hypertensive crisis, seizure prophylaxis/management (eclampsia tray).

All medications, consumables, and equipment for immediate resuscitation to manage convulsions or sudden maternal collapse should preferably be placed in a crash cart. Access to laboratory services and blood components and transfer facility to an obstetric ICU and HDU are to be ensured to dispense required care if patient becomes serious.

Q3. What should be the desired composition of the team required to deliver a patient of preeclampsia?

A team comprising a senior obstetrician, trained labor room nurses, a neonatologist with anesthetist on call and quick access to multidisciplinary team (intensivist, nephrologist, cardiologist, and hematologist) is recommended.

Q4. What should be the informed consent for delivery in a patient of preeclampsia?

Patient of preeclampsia is at high risk, it is advisable to explain about the condition with possible complications and obtain high risk consent as per presented on page 24 of Uniform consents provided by FOGSI 2020-2021.

Q5. What should be the baseline assessment of a patient of preeclampsia in labor?

All women with gestational hypertension or preeclampsia without severe features who are in labor must be monitored for early detection of progression to severe disease. They should be asked about premonitory symptoms of headache, feeling of discomfort, blurring of vision, vomiting, right upper quadrant pain, sudden excessive weight gain, and severe edema.

Blood pressure measurements, pulse, and symptom assessment are recommended. Clinical evaluation consists of per abdomen examination and pelvic assessment. It is advisable that investigations for CBC, platelets, coagulation profile, liver enzymes, BUN, LDH, and urine for proteinuria be ordered.

Clinical assessment of fetal well-being is done by fetal heart Doppler and reviewing available ultrasound report (for growth, weight, amniotic fluid volume, and Doppler).

If CTG is reactive and Bishop score is favorable, it can facilitate a vaginal birth with vigilant monitoring.

Timing of delivery: Decision to deliver should be carefully decided after assessing maternal and fetal risks.

Nonsevere preeclampsia: Pregnancy can be continued till term with vigilant monitoring and allowed spontaneous labor or induce after 37 completed weeks.

Severe preeclampsia: To be delivered after 34 completed weeks once mother is stabilized.

Eclampsia: Should be delivered once mother is stabilized after $MgSO_4$ and antihypertensives.

Labor induction with appropriate methods can be carried out safely in stabilized patients under close monitoring.

Cesarean section is done for obstetric indications.

Q6. How will you monitor a patient of preeclampsia in first stage of labor?

All patients of preeclampsia are to be monitored closely. It is recommended that the duration of labor should not be prolonged and follow the intrapartum care WHO guidelines.

Maternal monitoring:

Vital signs:

Blood pressure: Frequent monitoring, typically every 15–30 minutes during labor, depending on the severity of preeclampsia.

Pulse and respiratory rate and state of maternal hydration. Frequent monitoring to detect any signs of deterioration.

Neurological status: Regular assessments for symptoms such as headache, visual disturbances, and changes in mental status to detect early signs of eclampsia.

Fluid balance: Careful monitoring of fluid intake and output to avoid fluid overload and pulmonary edema is recommended. In women with severe preeclampsia, maintenance fluids limited to 80 mL/h. 1 mL/kg/h is beneficial unless there are other ongoing fluid losses. An additional 700 mL can be used for nonsensical loss. Crystalloids like Ringer's lactate or normal saline are recommended.

Indwelling catheter for accurate urine output is recommended in patients on magnesium sulfate.

Fetal monitoring: Vigilant monitoring of the fetus with continuous or intermittent Doppler device or electronic fetal heart monitoring is preferred, where available.

Progress of labor: Duration, frequency, and intensity of uterine contractions are to be monitored. Periodic vaginal examinations not earlier than 4 hours are recommended to assess changes in cervical effacement, dilatation rotation, and descent.

Maintaining and monitoring labor as per partogram is recommended to avoid prolonged labor.

Pain management: Epidural analgesia can be used where available and helps with pain management while also assisting in blood pressure control.

Q7. What are the indications for administering magnesium sulfate in labor?

Magnesium sulfate is the drug of choice for prevention and treatment of eclamptic seizures in women with severe preeclampsia. They are at a risk of seizures, intrapartum, as well as postpartum. It is recommended to use prophylactically, either Zuspan regimen, i.e., loading dose followed by IV maintenance or Pritchard regime, loading IV dose with intramuscular doses.

Patient needs to be monitored regularly for signs of toxicity of magnesium sulfate by assessing deep tendon reflexes (Patellar reflex), urine output, and respiratory rate.

Q8. What is the role of induction and augmentation of labor?

Induction and augmentation of labor are critical interventions in managing pregnancies complicated by preeclampsia. These interventions can help mitigate the risks associated with preeclampsia by ensuring timely delivery, thus preventing further complications for both mother and baby.

Induction of labor:
Role in preeclampsia: Induction of labor is often recommended to initiate delivery when the risks of continuing the pregnancy outweigh the benefits. This is especially important in preeclampsia, where delaying delivery can lead to severe complications such as eclampsia, HELLP syndrome, and placental abruption.

Induction of labor should be offered to mothers eligible for vaginal delivery. Prostaglandins (PGs) (dinoprostone gel, suppositories, or tablets) can be used for ripening. Misoprostol may be used in patients remote from term. Mechanical dilatation of the cervix with Foley's balloon or vaginal hygroscopic dilators may be considered.

Gestational age considerations: Induction is typically considered when the pregnancy reaches 37 weeks' gestation or earlier if severe features of preeclampsia are present (e.g., severe hypertension, organ dysfunction, or fetal compromise).

Reduction of maternal and fetal complications: Inducing labor can reduce the risk of maternal complications like stroke and organ failure, as well as fetal complications such as fetal growth restriction (FGR) and stillbirth.

In cases with severe preeclampsia and patient being stable, with a favorable Bishop score, induction of labor may reduce complications.

Augmentation of labor:
Role in preeclampsia: Enhancement of labor progress: Augmentation is used to strengthen and regulate contractions if labor is not progressing adequately. This can be particularly important in women with preeclampsia, where prolonged labor can increase risks of maternal and fetal distress. By ensuring efficient labor progress, augmentation can help reduce the likelihood of cesarean delivery, which carries additional risks in preeclampsia due to potential complications with anesthesia, bleeding, and recovery.

Oxytocin is the primary agent used for augmentation. It helps initiate and strengthen uterine contractions. It is used after amniotomy and checking color of grading of meconium.

Amniotomy: Artificial rupture of membranes can also be used to enhance labor progress.

Q9. How will you conduct the second stage of labor?

The second stage is conducted with close maternal and fetal monitoring and vaginal delivery is conducted as routine in an optimized/stable patient with restrictive use of episiotomy. Instrumental delivery is conducted as per obstetric indications.

Q10. How will you conduct the third stage of labor?

Active management of third stage of labor is recommended universally as per WHO guidelines to decrease PPH. All uterotonics can be safely used to manage uterine atony except Ergometrine (methylergonovine) which is known to precipitate hypertension due to vasoconstriction and can cause coronary spasm, myocardial ischemia, stroke, and seizures.

Q11. What are the indications of cesarean section (CS) in labor in patients with preeclampsia?

The decision to perform a cesarean section (CS) in preeclampsia and eclampsia is based on several factors.

Indications for cesarean section:
Maternal indications:

- Severe preeclampsia or eclampsia with unstable maternal condition irrespective of gestational age
- Failure to progress in labor with signs of maternal or fetal distress
- HELLP syndrome with significant thrombocytopenia or coagulopathy

Fetal indications:

- Nonreassuring fetal heart rate patterns indicating fetal distress
- Severe fetal growth restriction, with compromised fetal well-being fetal malpresentation

Anesthesia: Regional anesthesia (spinal or epidural) is preferred to reduce the risk of hypertensive complications, but general anesthesia may be required in emergencies with skilled anesthesia team.

Q12. How will you monitor the patient after birth and for how long?

Postpartum care is crucial in managing patients with preeclampsia and eclampsia, as complications can persist or arise after delivery.

Postpartum eclampsia is a known complication which can be prevented by continuing strict monitoring and medication for at least 48 hours after delivery.

Blood pressure monitoring:
Frequency: Regular monitoring of blood pressure in the immediate postpartum period and for at least 48 hours.

Antihypertensive therapy: Continuation and initiation of other antihypertensive medications as needed.

Magnesium sulfate:
Duration: Continued for 24 hours postpartum in women who had severe preeclampsia or eclampsia to prevent seizures beyond delivery or last convulsion whichever is later.

Monitoring for complications:
Symptoms: Watch for signs of persistent or new-onset symptoms such as severe headache, visual disturbances, epigastric pain, or shortness of breath.

Laboratory tests: Repeat tests for liver enzymes, kidney function, and platelet count if abnormalities were present antepartum.

Long-term follow-up:
Hypertension:

Persistence: Chronic hypertension may develop in some women, necessitating long-term management.

Follow-up: Regular follow-up visits to monitor blood pressure and assess the need for ongoing antihypertensive therapy.

Counseling:
- Contraception barrier, DMPA, and IUCD implants can be offered.
- *Future pregnancies:* Counseling on the risk of recurrence in future pregnancies and the importance of early prenatal care.
- *Cardiovascular health:* Education on the increased long-term risk of cardiovascular disease and lifestyle modifications to reduce this risk.
- *Lifestyle changes:* Weight control if high BMI, exercise, and healthy nutrition
- Availability of a functioning crash cart
- Though hypertensive disorders in pregnancy have been extensively reviewed, there is no single guideline to address intrapartum care in preeclampsia.
- Management of labor of each patient with preeclampsia has to be individualized with extreme caution and care. Country-specific good practice guidelines need to be drafted.

11

CHAPTER

Preeclampsia and the Heart

Palaniappan Narayanan

INTRODUCTION

Preeclampsia is a relatively common complication of pregnancy with a prevalence of 3–5%. It is showing a rising trend nowadays. It is the leading cause of morbidity and mortality for pregnant women and also has a significant economic burden on healthcare systems. The pathogenesis of PE may be different in nulliparous than that in women with preexisting vascular disease, multifetal gestation DM, or previous PE. In addition, the pathophysiologic abnormalities in the placenta of early onset PE may be different from that of an PE that develops near term, during labor or post-partum period.

It is a pregnancy-specific disorder with hypertension, leading on to multiorgan dysfunction. These effects are likely to persist even after pregnancy. Women with a history of preeclampsia are at increased risk for several non-communicable disorders, especially cardiovascular disease. The associations strengthen with repeated preeclampsia, fetal growth restriction, and preterm onset.

Since 2011, the American Heart Association (AHA) has recognized preeclampsia as a risk factor for cardiovascular disease (CVD) in women. In 2018, the AHA and the American College of Obstetricians and Gynecologists (ACOG) published a joint Presidential Advisory endorsing preeclampsia as a risk-enhancing factor that may direct statin initiation. ACOG recommends annual assessment of CVD risk factors for women with a history of recurrent or preterm preeclampsia.

PICO QUESTIONS WITH DRAFT RECOMMENDATIONS

Q1. Is there a relationship between preeclampsia and heart disease in women?

Ans. The possible future cardiovascular risks are cardiac failure, coronary heart disease, composite cardiovascular disease, death because of coronary artery disease.

Stroke and stroke death after preeclampsia

In preeclampsia, there is a two-fold increased risk of future coronary heart disease, and stroke. The risk for heart failure and death is increased four-fold.

The increase in the risk of heart failure, stroke, and cardiovascular disease death is higher during the first 10 years after a pregnancy affected by preeclampsia compared with that beyond 10 years.

In addition to a globally increased hazard of cardiovascular disease, a history of preeclampsia is also associated with 6–7 times increased risk of having recurrent ischemic attack within a year of developing acute coronary syndrome. Women with recurrent preeclampsia are characterized by a shorter life span (48.9 vs. 51.9 years), increased risk of ischemic heart disease (hazard ratio, 3.30), and stroke (hazard ratio, 5.10).

The estimation of cardiovascular disease risk and mortality differ in individual woman depending on the severity as well as type of HDP. The more severe form is associated with higher risk of CVD.

Q2. What are the common risk factors for preeclampsia and CVD?

Ans. Factors that predispose women to preeclampsia are also found in the risk profile for cardiovascular diseases. These include obesity, metabolic abnormalities, dyslipidemia, insulin resistance, heightened inflammatory responses, hypercoagulable states, and endothelial dysfunction.

Q3. Is pregnancy a cardiometabolic stress?

Ans. Pregnancy is a metabolic and vascular "stress test" for women in the same way that it is a metabolic stress test for future development of diabetes. Those who "fail" are at a higher risk for long-term cardiovascular complications. All the more if a woman develops preeclampsia or other manifestations of placental dysfunction, she is at greater risk to develop coronary heart disease, stroke, and cardiovascular disease. The risk is highest in women who develop both maternal (e.g., hypertension and proteinuria) and fetal (e.g., intrauterine growth restriction, preterm delivery) manifestations of abnormal placentation. The shared prepregnancy risk factors for both preeclampsia and cardiovascular diseases such as obesity, diabetes, dyslipidemia, socioeconomic, and behavioral factors, may also be the reason for the association between CVD and preeclampsia.

It is also possible that PE induces increased inflammatory mediators, endothelial dysfunction, sympathetic overactivity, insulin resistance, left ventricular hypertrophy and abnormal lipid profile leading to CVD. However more research is needed regarding the use of pregnancy history in CVD risk prediction and risk reduction intervention as many studies observed that association of CVD is not statistically significant when adjusted for established risk factors.

In addition, PE is a known risk factor for cardiomyopathy both peripartum and years after giving birth. women with PE have increased risk of cardiomyopathy for >5 years after giving birth than in general population.

Q4. Is preeclampsia an independent risk factor for early onset CVD?

Ans. The hemodynamic changes during pregnancy are well understood. There is a progressive increase in cardiac output and a decline in the systemic vascular resistance. This leads to a high-volume, low-resistance circulation. These changes peak in the middle of third trimester. Later cardiac output falls and systemic vascular resistance increases toward 40 weeks gestation. In uncomplicated normal pregnancies echocardiographic studies show an excessive increase in the left ventricular mass and remodeling with associated diastolic dysfunction in a small but significant proportion of women at term. All of these changes revert to normal postpartum. That is the reason why, pregnancy has been described as a stress test which unmasks women who have poor cardiovascular reserve or dysfunction.

In preeclamptic women maternal echocardiography studies have demonstrated significant cardiac dysfunction both before and at clinical manifestation of preeclampsia.

That cardiac output was significantly lower in early onset (<34 weeks) preeclampsia compared with late (>34 weeks). Preeclampsia was demonstrated by Valensie et al. A recent systematic review summarizing 36 studies of maternal cardiovascular function among 815 women with preeclampsia, demonstrated that increased vascular resistance and left ventricular mass were the most consistent findings of preeclampsia. Left ventricular wall thickness of >1.0 cm, exaggerated reduction in early diastole/atrial contraction, and lateral e' of <14 cm/s which are markers of diastolic dysfunction seen in preeclampsia are the differentiating features from normal pregnancy. Diastolic dysfunction and left ventricular remodeling are most marked in severe- and early-onset preeclampsia.

A study done by (B Thilaganathan) states cardiac maladaptation in term pregnancies with PE demonstrate significant subclinical myocardial changes on spectral tracking analysis.

It is associated with poor maternal and fetal outcomes, irrespective of the conventional classification of preeclampsia based on clinical severity or gestation of onset. These echo findings demonstrate that even apparently normal pregnancy shows significant strain on the maternal cardiovascular system. In women with evidence of worsening cardiovascular maladaptation, preeclampsia is the recognized clinical phenotype.

Several mediators of endothelial cell dysfunction are up regulated in preeclampsia as in cardiovascular disorders. Free radical derived oxidative stress, leukocyte adhesion, various inflammatory markers, including neutrophil response, C-reactive protein, may contribute to endothelial dysfunction in both preeclampsia and coronary atherosclerosis. Even preeclampsia itself can induce metabolic and vascular changes which may increase the overall future risk for CVD in affected women.

Nevertheless, clinicians should discuss the link between PE and future cardio vascular risk and be more aggressive about healthy life style and behavior such as extended lactation, weight loss, BMI, smoking cessation, regular balanced diet, and motivation to reduce modifiable risk factors, they should be closely followed and treated for modifiable CVD risk factors aggressively.

Pathogenesis CVD in Preeclampsia

It is well established that there is a relationship between placental dysfunction and cardiovascular diseases and the main pathology in preeclampsia defective vascularization of placenta. The stress signals from the dysfunctional placenta to the cardiovascular system of mother can aggravate cardiovascular dysfunction and thereby predispose to cardiovascular disease to occur prematurely. Women with recurrent preeclampsia have increased carotid intima-media thickness and peak mitral filling early diastole/atrial contraction ratio, and lower cardiac output and left ventricular mass, compared to women with a normal follow-on pregnancy.

In a landmark study, Romundstad et al. assessed whether the predisposition of preeclamptic women to increased risk for cardiovascular disease later in life can be attributed to pregnancy factors or to prepregnancy risk factors that are shared by both disorders. The results of Romundstad et al. suggested that the positive association of preeclampsia to postpartum cardiovascular risk is mainly due to shared prepregnancy risk factors rather than reflecting a direct influence of preeclamptic pregnancy on the maternal cardiovascular system. That all of these risk factors are also known to be correlated with cardiovascular morbidity in nonpregnant adults is consistent with the hypothesis that poor cardiovascular reserve predisposes to the placentally mediated disorder of preeclampsia **(Fig. 1)**.

Preeclampsia is an independent risk factor for early onset coronary artery calcification.

Recently studies are coming up, showing preeclampsia as an independent risk factor for CVD. Obviously, preeclampsia is a sex-specific cardiovascular risk enhancer. It is associated with premature CVD such as stroke and myocardial infarction. Benschop et al. showed that preeclampsia is an independent risk factor for early onset coronary artery calcification (CAC) in young women. Those with prior preeclampsia ages 45–50 years were four times as likely to have CAC compared to women ages 40–45.

The most significant difference in CAC between women with and without a history of preeclampsia was seen in women ages 40–45 years (23% vs. 10%; $p = 0.003$). Women with a history of preeclampsia ages 45–50 years were four times as likely to have some CAC compared to women ages 40–45 years (OR 4.3, 95% CI 1.5–12.2). after adjusting for covariates such as smoking status,

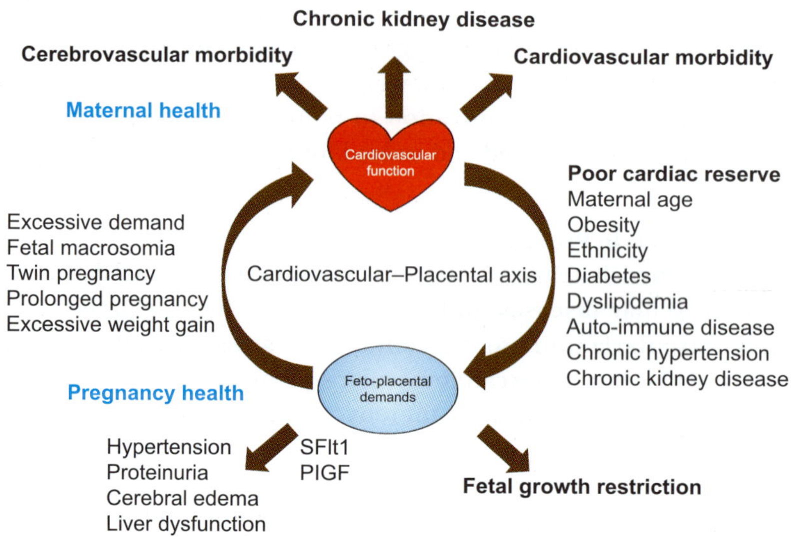

Fig. 1: Diagram illustrating the interaction between maternal cardiovascular function and placental function, maternal health, and fetal well-being. Placental oxidative stress or hypoxia is related to the relative balance of cardiovascular functional reserve and the cardiovascular volume/resistance load of pregnancy. The final common pathway that results in the signs and symptoms of preeclampsia involves the release of placental vasoactive substances. PIGF indicates placenta growth factor; and sFLT, soluble fms-like tyrosine kinase.

BMI, diabetes, hypertension, and hyperlipidemia. The Framingham Risk Score (FRS) was higher for women with a history of preeclampsia in each age group, whereas only the 55–63-year-old age group had a FRS >10%, meeting current guidelines for preventive treatment. Though women with preeclampsia appear to have increased risk for traditional cardiovascular risk factors (hypertension ,smoking, diabetes, obesity, and hyperlipidemia) to explain increased incidence of CVD, preeclampsia is an independent risk factor for early onset CAC and subclinical CVD.

A history of preeclampsia in pregnancy has previously been associated with an increased risk of CAC 30 years post-pregnancy, after controlling for traditional risk factors. This new study by Benschop et al. is the first study to shed light on the timing of early onset subclinical CVD in women with a history of preeclampsia.

While much of the increased risk of CVD associated with a history of preeclampsia appears to be mediated through traditional CVD risk factors such as chronic hypertension or obesity that arise in the years or decades after pregnancy, some 20–40% of the excess CVD risk associated with preeclampsia history is not explained by conventional risk factors. Moreover, even when it predicts later-developing CVD risk factors, preeclampsia remains an early warning sign of future CVD risk, predicting a doubling of CVD risk before the traditional CVD risk factors emerge. This fact helps women as well as clinicians a longer time to implement lifestyle changes which are known to reduce risk even among this high-risk group.

Q5. What are the risk modulation strategies to reduce CVD after preeclampsia?

Ans. With various revisions of the classifications of hypertensive disorders of pregnancy (HDP), the task force on hypertension. The four categories of hypertensive disorders in pregnancy specified by ACOG in 2013 are preeclampsia-eclampsia, chronic hypertension, chronic hypertension with superimposed preeclampsia, and gestational hypertension.

The risk modulation of this enigmatic disease lies in the understanding of its mysterious pathogenesis, while various theories are put forth the oxidative stress at the fetomaternal interface, immune mechanism, and angiogenic factors play a pivotal role. The levels of PIGF, sFlt1, and sEng and the ratios of sFLT1 to PIGF and PIGF to sEng, vary grossly between preeclampsia and normotensive women.

Hence, the risk modulation of this disease is based on the use of proteomic studies using protein microarray, mass spectrometry, urinary proteomics and metabolomics, and hence we can use novel therapy as strategies in the risk modulation of their disease.

sFlt1 Ligands

VEGF is a natural ligand for sFlt 1 and recombinant VEGF2, is a novel non-heparin binding form of VEGF and hence has been proved as a therapy for preeclampsia in pregnant mice infusion of VEGF 121 lowers blood pressure in a uterine pressure model of preeclampsia in rats.

RNA interference-based strategies

Scientists discovered novel RNAi with molecules which specifically target all of the major sFLT, mRNAs in cell culture studies. They also demonstrated that a single dose of sFLT1 RNAi given intravenously reduced the sFLT, protein level by 50%, which was associated with a lowering in blood pressure and proteinuria in preeclamptic baboons. In low resource countries with high incidence of preeclampsia the cost of production of oligonucleotide therapy would be definitely less expensive than that of recombinant proteins.

Small Molecule Inhibitors

Various small molecules inhibitors such as sildenafil citrate, ouabain, metformin, esomeprazole, were used in various studies in a hope to reduce hypertension and its sequalae but could not be proved with definite incidence owing to varying results.

Apheresis

Removing excess antiangiogenic proteins with extracorporeal methods is a good therapeutic strategy for preeclampsia as it arouses exposure of the fetus to harmful drugs. Thadani and Ananth S Karumanchi et al. used a dextran-sulfate apheresis (DSA) column which was marketed for LDL removal to reduce sFLT 1 through interactions between the negatively charged DSA and the positively charged sFLT1 proteins. They reported this treatment safe in women with preterm preeclampsia (<32 weeks), including lowering of proteinuria, decreased blood pressure, and prolonging gestation. This may be a novel technique in future to reduce risk categorization and modulation in women with HDP.

Aspirin

The use of low-dose aspirin (LDA) as a strategy to reduce risks in preeclampsia had been used for years starting from the CLASP (collaborative low dose aspirin study in pregnancy) to the recent ASPRE trial. Aspirin at a dose of 150 mg per day led to a 62% reduction in preterm preeclampsia compared with a placebo. After the enormous evidence the usage of aspirin started at ≥16 weeks of gestation to 34 weeks, has almost become the panacea for prevention of preeclampsia and its sequelae.

Statins

Statins are competitive inhibitors of the enzyme 5(OH) 3-CH3 glutaryl COA reductase (HMG COA reductase), which is the rate controlling step in cholesterol synthesis. Pravastatin is a first-generation statin which is the most hydrophilic, hepatoselective and weak inhibitor of HMG COA reductase.

Constantine et al. used 10 mg of pravastatin which reduced the rate of PE and preterm delivery without any increased risk for mother and fetus.

Statins have shown to improve vascular function via stimulating HOI expression and hence leading to enhanced NO synthetase and decreased placental production of sFLT1. Pravastatin is the mostly commonly studied drug in anti-phospholipid antibody syndrome, the STAMP trial of pravastatin in early onset preeclampsia also threw a little light. Further better studies are required to comment on the role of statins in preventing preeclampsia.

The INOVASIA trial randomized participants to pravastatin (2 × 20 mg oral daily) in addition to the standard regimen of aspirin 80 mg and calcium 1 g from 14 to 20 weeks until delivery versus aspirin and calcium alone. The pravastatin group had lower rates of PE (13.8% vs. 26.7%) and preterm delivery <39 weeks (16.1% vs. 36%).

Statins were initially classified as category X by the FDA due to theoretic concern for teratogenic effects and lack of indications to use in pregnancy. But recent data and use in pregnancy has created more evidence. Although statins decrease maternal cholesterol levels, no effect on fetal cholesterol levels and fetal weight with the use of pravastatin in pregnancy. So, in July 2021, the FDA removed the strongest warning against the use of statins in pregnancy.

Research Gaps: The very idea of the heart as a central organ for preeclampsia is new, and the research gaps are huge and evidence is limited and there are lots of research gaps.

CONCLUSION

Preeclampsia per se as well as because of its shared risk factors with CVD, has a high chance of future cardiovascular risk. Therefore, pregnancy should be viewed as the window for future cardiovascular diseases occurrence and early opportunity to intervene with steps aimed at preventing or delaying later CVD risk factors and events. The severe the preeclampsia, the greater the chance of developing CVD in future. The investigation for selective biomarkers that may prospectively signal identify women who will develop cardiac disease is an exciting area of study and future possibility to improve lives of women around the world.

Preeclampsia used to be recognized by its severity, then according to the gestation of onset. In future, cardiovascular phenotyping of PE is likely to prove more clinically useful. Whether it is prudent to recommend an echocardiography for all pregnancies as screening tool and if so at what gestational age is not too sure.

We need to focus on better postnatal cardiovascular assessment after preeclampsia. preventive counseling more vigilant screening and management of modifiable risk factors should be provided to the affected.

Clinicians should closely monitor in the first 3 years postpartum and continuously for two decades so that we will not miss the opportunity to alter the disease course.

- Preeclampsia is associated with increased future risk of cardiovascular diseases, such as CAD and stroke.
- Recent studies show preeclampsia itself as an independent risk factor for future CVD and can be attributed to underlying genetic factors and risk factors that are common to both preeclampsia and CVD.
- Evidence shows a strong relationship between recurrent preeclampsia and additional risk of developing CVD, diabetes, dyslipidemia, congestive heart failure, and cerebrovascular disease later in life when compared to single pregnancy with preeclampsia.
- Risk stratification and prevention plays an important role in reducing CVD and mortality.
- Integrated efforts of patients, care givers, researchers, and national organizations are required to improve CVD prevention.

BIBLIOGRAPHY

1. Aldika Akbar MI, Azis MA, Riu DS, et al. INOVASIA Study: A Multicenter Randomized Clinical Trial of Pravastatin to Prevent Preeclampsia in High-Risk Patients. Am J Perinatol. 2024.
2. American College of Obstetricians and Gynaecologists. Hypertension in pregnancy. Report of the American College of Obstetricians and Gynecologists' Task Force on Hypertension in Pregnancy. Obstet Gynecol. 2013;122(5):1122-31.
3. Benschop L, Brouwers L, Zoet GA, et al. Early onset of coronary artery calcification in women with previous preeclampsia. Circ Cardiovasc Imaging. 2020;13:e010340.
4. Brown HL, Warner JJ, Gianos E, et al. Promoting risk identification and reduction of cardiovascular disease in women through collaboration with obstetricians and gynecologists: A presidential advisory from the American Heart Association and the American College of Obstetricians and Gynecologists. Circulation. 2018;137:e843-52.
5. Castleman JS, Ganapathy R, Taki F, et al. Echocardiographic structure and function in hypertensive disorders of pregnancy: a systematic review. Circ Cardiovasc Imaging. 2016;9:e004888.
6. Charkiewicz K, Jasinska E, Laudanski P. Identification of proteomic biomarkers of preeclampsia using protein microarray and tandem mass spectrometry [Polish]. Postepy Hig Med Dosw. 2015;69:562-70.
7. Dall'Asta A, D'Antonio F, Saccone G, et al. Cardiovascular events following pregnancy complicated by pre-eclampsia with emphasis on comparison between early- and late-onset forms: systematic review and meta-analysis. Ultrasound Obstet Gynecol. 2021;57(5):698-709.
8. Ghossein-Doha C, van Neer J, Wissink B, et al. Pre-eclampsia: an important risk factor for asymptomatic heart failure. Ultrasound Obstet Gynecol. 2017;49:143-9.
9. Gilbert JS, Verzwyvelt J, Colson D, et al. Recombinant vascular endothelial growth factor 121 infusion lowers blood pressure and improves renal function in rats with placental ischemia-induced hypertension. Hypertension. 2010;55:380-5.
10. Grand'Maison S, Pilote L, Schlosser K, et al. Clinical features and outcomes of acute coronary syndrome in women with previous pregnancy complications. Can J Cardiol. 2017;33:1683-92.
11. Kalafat E, Sukur YE, Abdi A, et al. Metformin for the prevention of hypertensive disorders of pregnancy in women with gestational diabetes and obesity: a systematic review and meta-analysis. Ultrasound Obstet Gynecol. 2018;52:706-14.
12. Kleinrouweler CE, Wiegerinck MM, Ris-Stalpers C, et al. Accuracy of circulating placental growth factor, vascular endothelial growth factor, soluble fms-like tyrosine kinase 1 and soluble endoglin in the prediction of pre-eclampsia: a systematic review and meta-analysis. BJOG. 2012;119:778-87.
13. Krasne M, Wand A, Park K, et al. Preeclampsia is an Independent Risk Factor for Early Onset Coronary Artery Calcification: A Call for Risk Assessment and Modification. Am Coll Cardiol. 2021.
14. Leaños-Miranda A, Campos-Galicia I, Isordia-Salas I, et al. Changes in circulating concentrations of soluble fms-like tyrosine kinase-1 and placental growth factor measured by automated electrochemiluminescence immunoassays methods are predictors of preeclampsia. J Hypertens. 2012;30:2173-81.

15. Lefkou E, Mamopoulos A, Dagklis T, et al. Pravastatin improves pregnancy outcomes in obstetric antiphospholipid syndrome refractory to antithrombotic therapy. J Clin Invest. 2016;126:2933-40.
16. Melchiorre K, Sharma R, Khalil A, et al. Maternal cardiovascular function in normal pregnancy: evidence of maladaptation to chronic volume overload. Hypertension. 2016;67:754-62.
17. Mosca L, Benjamin EJ, Berra K, et al. Effectiveness-based guidelines for the prevention of cardiovascular disease in women—2011 update: A guideline from the American Heart Association. Circulation 2011;123:1243-62.
18. Paauw ND, Terstappen F, Ganzevoort W, et al. Sildenafil during pregnancy: a preclinical meta-analysis on fetal growth and maternal blood pressure. Hypertension. 2017;70:998-1006.
19. Park K, Wu P, Gulati M. Obstetrics and gynecological history: a missed opportunity for cardiovascular risk assessment. J Am Coll Cardiol Case Rep. 2020;2:161-63.
20. Ramma W, Ahmed A. Therapeutic potential of statins and the induction of heme oxygenase-1 in preeclampsia. J Reprod Immunol. 2014;101-02, 153-60.
21. Rana S, Rajakumar A, Geahchan C, et al. Ouabain inhibits placental sFlt1 production by repressing HSP27-dependent HIF-1alpha pathway. FASEB J. 2014;28:4324-34.
22. Rolnik DL, Wright D, Poon LC, et al. Aspirin versus placebo in pregnancies at high risk for preterm preeclampsia. N Engl J Med. 2017;377:613-22.
23. Romundstad PR, Magnussen EB, Smith GD, et al. Hypertension in Pregnancy and Later Cardiovascular Risk: Common Antecedents? Circulation. 2010;122(6):579-84.
24. Savu O, Jurcuţ R, Giuşcă S, et al. Morphological and functional adaptation of the maternal heart during pregnancy. Circ Cardiovasc Imaging. 2012;5:289-97.
25. Sep SJ, Schreurs MP, Bekkers SC, et al. Early-pregnancy changes in cardiac diastolic function in women with recurrent pre-eclampsia and in previously pre-eclamptic women without recurrent disease. BJOG. 2011;118:1112-9.
26. Staff AC, Redman CW, Williams D, et al. Pregnancy and long-term maternal cardiovascular health: progress through harmonization of research cohorts and biobanks. Hypertension. 2016;67:251-60.
27. Stergiotou I, Bijnens B, Cruz-Lemini M, et al. Maternal subclinical vascular changes in fetal growth restriction with and without pre-eclampsia. Ultrasound Obstet Gynecol. 2015;46:706-12.
28. Thadhani R, Kisner T, Hagmann H, et al. Pilot study of extracorporeal removal of soluble fms-like tyrosine kinase 1 in preeclampsia. Circulation. 2011;124:940-50.
29. Turanov AA, Lo A, Hassler MR, et al. RNAi modulation of placental sFLT1 for the treatment of preeclampsia. Nat. Biotechnol. 2018;36:1164-73.
30. Valensise H, Vasapollo B, Gagliardi G, et al. Early and late preeclampsia: two different maternal hemodynamic states in the latent phase of the disease. Hypertension. 2008;52:873-80.
31. Wu P, Haththotuwa R, Kwok CS, et al. A Systematic Review and Meta-Analysis. Circ Cardiovasc Qual Outcomes. 2017;10(2):e003497.

12 CHAPTER

Complications of Preeclampsia and their Management

12.1 ECLAMPSIA

S Sampathkumari

Q1. What are premonitory signs and clinical features of eclampsia?

Draft recommendations:

Premonitory signs of eclampsia are:

- Persistent occipital or frontal headaches
- Visual disturbances like blurred vision, photophobia, diplopia, scotoma, photopsia (flashes of light in the field of vision)
- Altered mental status
- Epigastric pain
- Nausea and vomiting

Eclampsia is described as the occurrence of one or more tonic-clonic convulsions in a widespread manner in pregnant women with hypertension disorders that are unrelated to other medical diseases.

Summary of evidence:

- It is estimated that 78–83% cases of eclampsia are often preceded by premonitory signs.
- It is believed that headaches are a sign of developing cerebral edema, hypertensive encephalopathy, and high cerebral perfusion pressure. However, eclampsia can occur in the absence of warning signs or symptoms.

It is observed that:

- 59–70% of seizures will happen in the antepartum period.
- 20–30% during labor
- 20–30% during the postpartum phase.

Q2. What is the immediate management for stabilizing eclampsia?

Draft recommendations:

During or immediately after the acute convulsive episode, supportive care should be given to prevent serious maternal injury.

This includes:

- Establishing airway patency

- Ensuring oxygenation
- Avoiding aspiration

During this time, the bedside rails should be elevated and padded. The patient should lie in the lateral decubitus position and have oral secretions suctioned when required to reduce the risk of aspiration.

Summary of evidence:

- Even though the first seizure normally passes within few minutes, it is crucial to keep the patient oxygenated by administering extra oxygen through a facemask at a rate of 8–10 L/min. Pulse oximeter is used for monitoring maternal oxygen saturation.
- Only in the event that the pulse oximetry readings are abnormal (oxygen saturation of 92%), will arterial blood gas analysis be necessary

Q3. What is stepwise further management of eclampsia?

Draft recommendations:

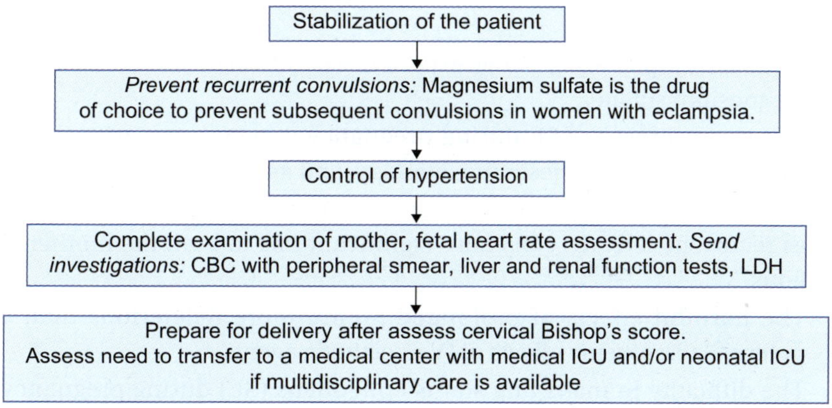

Summary of evidence:

- The presence of eclampsia would be an indication for delivery, although it is not an indication for cesarean delivery.
- The mode of delivery should be assessed based on cervical Bishop's score, gestational age, fetal conditions.
- When the maternal conditions stabilize and patient is conscious alert and oriented to time and place induction of labor can be done.
- Induction of labor is reasonable as long as the patient is in active labor within 24 hours.
- Women with eclampsia should have close monitoring of their vital signs, intake, output, and symptoms for a minimum of 72 hours following delivery.

Q4. How do you manage recurrent, refractory seizures, and status eclampticus management?

Draft recommendations:

- *Recurrent eclampsia:* In such a scenario, an additional intravenous (IV) bolus of 2 g magnesium sulfate may be administered over a period of 3–5 minutes.
- Refractory seizure (seizing at 20 minutes after the bolus or more than two recurrences), sodium amobarbital (250 mg IV in 3 minutes), thiopental, or phenytoin (1,250 mg IV at a rate of 50 mg/minute) can be given.
- Status epilepticus is a single epileptic seizure lasting more than 5 min or two or more seizures occurring within a 5-minute period without the person returning to normal between them.
- The first-line agent for treatment of SE was lorazepam and midazolam.
- Levetiracetam and phenobarbitone are the most suitable second-line agents.
- IV anesthetic agents that can be used are propofol and thiopentone.

Summary of evidence:

- 10% of eclamptic women may experience another convulsion after taking magnesium sulfate.
- The management of SE during pregnancy depends on various factors such as the period of gestation, etiology, and associated comorbidities.
- In general, termination of pregnancy is the rule in cases of refractory SE, as recurrent seizures can cause significant risk to both the mother and fetus.
- The harmful effects of prolonged SE are more deleterious than the potential teratogenic effects of IV anesthetic agents.
- The difficulty in managing status epilepticus (SE) during pregnancy is in controlling the seizures quickly while keeping in mind the safety and tolerability of anesthetics and antiepileptic medications.

Q5. What are complications of eclampsia?

Draft recommendations: Women with eclampsia have increased risk of severe maternal complications like:

- Placental abruption
- HELLP
- Disseminated intravascular coagulation
- Pulmonary edema
- Aspiration pneumonia
- Cardiopulmonary arrest
- Acute renal failure

Summary of evidence:

- Referrals to tertiary care centers are necessary for women who have eclampsia remote from term.
- Blood pressure must be stabilized and convulsions must be under control before transferring an eclamptic patient to a tertiary care center.
- A loading dose of magnesium sulfate should be administered to the patient, and fetal monitoring should be started.
- In order to ensure appropriate therapy in the event of further convulsions, patients ought to be transported in an ambulance with medical personnel present.

Q6. What is differential diagnosis of eclampsia?

Draft recommendations:

There may be overlap between eclampsia's clinical presentation and symptoms and various medical and surgical diseases.

Alternative diagnoses should be considered in the following scenarios:

- Normal blood pressures with absence of proteinuria
- Focal neurologic deficits
- Onset before 20 weeks of gestation or >48 hours after delivery
- Prolonged loss of consciousness

Differential diagnosis of seizure during pregnancy or after delivery:
Pregnancy related:

- Eclampsia
- Thrombotic thrombocytopenic purpura
- Amniotic fluid emboli

Neovascular:

- Intracranial hemorrhage
- Subarachnoid hemorrhage
- Arterial embolism or thrombosis
- Angiomas
- Space occupying lesion of the brain (benign or neoplastic)
- Posterior reversible encephalopathy syndrome
- Congenital brain defects

Metabolic causes:

- Liver or renal failure
- Hypoglycemia
- Hyponatremia
- Hyperosmolar states
- Hypocalcemia

Autoimmune:

- Systemic lupus erythematosus
- Antiphospholipid syndrome

Infectious meningitis or encephalitis

Drug or substance overdose or withdrawal (e.g., tricyclic antidepressants, benzodiazepines, salicylate overdose)

Trauma

Psychogenic nonepileptic seizures

For additional evaluation, brain imaging with an MRI or CT scan should be performed. Etiological distinction is important since therapy needs to target the underlying condition.

Summary of evidence:

- For most clinicians, the diagnosis of eclampsia is evident when a woman arrives with convulsions, proteinuria, and hypertension. Even though hypertension is a defining feature of eclampsia, it may not be present in as many as 25% of cases.
- If an alternative diagnosis is considered, the path toward the diagnosis of a seizure in pregnant women will begin with a thorough history and physical examination.
- Evaluation of the underlying causes is necessary.
- These may include drug misuse, medical comorbidities, and medication.

Q7. What are effects of eclampsia on neonate?

Draft recommendations:

Neonates of women with eclampsia are at increased risk of:

- Small for gestational age (SGA)
- Complications related to prematurity such as respiratory distress syndrome and neonatal death.

Summary of evidence:

High rates of perinatal mortality and morbidity persist in pregnancies with eclampsia. The range of the reported perinatal death rate is 5.6–11.8%. Fetal growth limitation, placental abruption, or extreme preterm are the main causes of perinatal deaths.

Q8. What is the risk of recurrence in future pregnancies?

Draft recommendations:

- Pregnant women with a history of eclampsia are more likely to develop preeclampsia.

- Preeclampsia occurs in roughly 25% of subsequent pregnancies, and the risk is increased if eclampsia first appeared in the second trimester of pregnancy.
- Recurrent eclampsia occurs at a rate of roughly 2%.
- A 12-fold higher risk of cardiovascular morbidity, including myocardial infarction, cerebrovascular illness, acute heart failure, cardiomyopathy, or cardiac arrest, was linked to eclampsia.

Summary of evidence: Women who suffered eclampsia may report long-term cognitive difficulties related to memory and concentration after the pregnancy. Women who had multiple eclamptic seizures report greater cognitive decline than women who experience 1epsiode of eclampsia.

Q9. Describe APLA and eclampsia.

Draft recommendations:

- The prevalence of APLA in women experiencing obstetrical problems can reach 5–40%.
- Thrombotic events are caused by antiphospholipid antibodies (APLAs), which are mostly targeted against phospholipid-binding proteins.
- Lupus anticoagulant, anticardiolipin (anti-CL) antibodies, and anti-β_2-Glycoprotein 1 (anti-β_2GP1) antibodies are examples of APLAs.

These antibodies are part of the diagnostic criteria for antiphospholipid syndrome (APS) and are typical markers of the condition.

Modified Sapporo criteria is used for diagnosing antiphospholipid antibody syndrome.

Summary of evidence:

- The mechanism that is proposed is the infarction of placental blood vessels due to placental thrombotic events. Abruption, decidual arteriopathy in small placentas, infarctions in the core parts of the placenta, and intervillous thrombosis are common pathological characteristics.
- A diverse class of autoantibodies known as antiphospholipid antibodies (APLAs) are focused on attacking either anionic (cardiolipin, phosphatidylserine) or phospholipids that are neutral (phosphatidylethanolamine) as well as plasma that binds phospholipids.
- Preeclampsia and eclampsia are among the most threatening conditions seen in APLA positive patient becoming pregnant.
- Analyzing the APLAs profiles in every woman with obstetric APS, which enables the evaluation of pregnancy risk and allows to monitor of the potential benefits of antithrombotic treatment, which gives the best effect if started in the first trimester.
- Preeclampsia and eclampsia are among the most threatening conditions seen in APLA positive patient becoming pregnant.

12.2 PREECLAMPSIA AND APH

Sareena Gilvaz

Q1. Antepartum hemorrhage (APH) and preeclampsia (PE): Is there a common pathophysiological mechanism between PE and abruption?

In women with chronic hypertension the risk of developing abruptio is 3–4-fold higher and with preeclampsia the risk of developing abruptio is 4–6-fold higher especially so when PE is associated with its severe features or it is superimposed over chronic hypertension.

The pathophysiology of abruption involves long drawn chronic issues along with acute triggers in the form of thrombosis, inflammation, infection in association with decidual and uteroplacental vasculopathy. This gives rise to placental hypo-perfusion and defective spiral artery remodeling, placental infarction and shallow trophoblastic invasion, all causing relative hypoxia and its associated expression of the vascular endothelial growth factors which is likely to affect the inflammatory response thus predisposing to abruptio and other similar placental mediated issues such as FGR and PE. This can occur several weeks and months before these events clinically manifest.

These clinical processes when associated with vascular reactivity, platelet activation and oxidative stress all lead to utero-placental ischemia same as that seen in preeclampsia which increases the risk of placental abruption.

Thus we see a common pathophysiology namely for placentation and utero placental under perfusion collectively called ischemic placental disease

The common pathophysiology thus being that they both share a uteroplacental ischemia and when there is a chronic pathology as stated above it only requires an acute trigger before it manifests itself. Thus we see that these 2 clinical conditions have a common underlying factor.

Q2. Can placental abruption in a prior pregnancy cause PE in a subsequent pregnancy and what is the association with preterm abruptio and PE?

Yes, placental abruption in a prior pregnancy can cause preeclampsia in a subsequent pregnancy and this is more so when it is a prior pre term abruptio. This observation has been validated and the reason quoted being that preterm abruptios are more associated with utero placental ischemia. The above fact was proved by a population based case control study done in Finland between 1996–2010. Preterm abruptio described as that which occurred before 37 weeks of gestation. They inferred that preterm abruption was associated with over a twofold increase in risk of preeclampsia (OR 2.2, 95% CI 1.5, 3.3 as compared to term abruptio which was not associated with preeclampsia (OR 1.1, 95 % CI 0.7. 1.7).

We also see that when there is a history of preterm abruptio along with preeclampsia, this increased the risk of preeclampsia developing in a subsequent pregnancy to as much as 16 fold, thereby, telling us that there is biological interaction between these two conditions.

Q3. Is there a relationship between maternal thrombophilia and the occurrence of preeclampsia and abruption?

Maternal thrombophilias (primary and acquired) have shown an association with placental abruption. In a systematic review Robertson at al showed in over 7 studies the association with thrombophilias and placental abruption. And this was more so with the heterozygous factor V Leiden (OR 4.70, 95% CI 1.13–19.59) and heterozygous prothrombin 20210A (OR 7.71, 95% CI 3.01–19.76).

Though thus said, a recent systematic review and meta-analysis of prospective cohort studies have questioned this above association and hence until further studies come to validate the above statement it still stands questionable.

Q4. Can reduction of high BP reduce incidence of abruptio and can be avoid the development of abruption?

One of main risk factors of abruptio placenta is hypertensive disorder of pregnancy whether it be chronic hypertension or gestational hypertension. That said, in a manner of speaking reduction in BP should potentially reduce the development of placental abruptio. The reason stated being reduction of blood pressure would reduce the stress on blood vessels including that of the placenta, thus, lowering the incidence of its premature separation.

However, this is a complex process as it involves the severity of hypertension, its other associated risk factors along with the timing and prompt but gradual mode of BP reduction. Thus close monitoring of BP and timely delivery would be the essence of management.

12.3 HELLP SYNDROME

Komal N Chavan

INTRODUCTION

- HELLP syndrome is a rare, potentially life-threatening obstetric complication characterized by hemolysis, elevated liver enzyme concentrations, and low platelet count.
- It is widely considered to represent a severe form of severe preeclampsia; however, the relationship between disorders is controversial, and some consider HELLP syndrome a separate disorder.
- Typically develops in the third trimester of pregnancy or early postpartum period and, in most cases, is preceded by hypertension and proteinuria.

- Presentation can be variable, and symptoms are often nonspecific; right upper quadrant or epigastric pain, nausea, vomiting, and headache are common.
- Diagnosis is based on the presence of microangiopathic hemolytic anemia on peripheral blood smear; elevated liver enzyme concentrations, specifically AST more than 2 times upper reference range for local laboratory (usually 70 units/L or higher) and thrombocytopenia (typical cutoff is less than 100,000/mm^3); usually in conjunction with hypertension and proteinuria.
- Delivery is the only effective method of treatment, severity of the condition and fetal condition.
- Immediate delivery after maternal stabilization is indicated in pregnancies at 34 weeks' of gestation or longer, less than 23–24 weeks' gestation, and between 23 and 34 weeks of gestation if there is disseminated intravascular coagulation, liver infarction or hemorrhage, renal failure, pulmonary edema, suspected abruptio placentae, or nonreassuring fetal status.
- Delivery can be delayed for 24 to 48 hours to allow administration of corticosteroid to assist fetal lung maturation in pregnancies between 23 and 34 weeks of gestation, providing patient and fetal conditions remain stable.
- Route of delivery is selected primarily on maternal condition, level of the platelets and also on basis of gestational age, fetal presentation, cervical status, obstetric history, and patient and fetal condition.
- Early diagnosis and appropriate management will get better Prognosis for both patient and the fetus. Although serious complications are common, perinatal morbidity and mortality is primarily caused by early gestational age at delivery.
- HELLP syndrome requires immediate obstetric consultation, patient stabilization, and delivery of fetus within 48 hours.

Q1. What is the prevalence of HELLP syndrome in preeclampsia?

HELLP syndrome is a rare, potentially life-threatening obstetric complication; characterized by hemolysis, elevated liver enzyme concentrations, and a low platelet count.

Occurs in 0.5% to 0.9% of all pregnancies and in 10–20% of patients with severe preeclampsia.

It may represent a complication or progression of severe preeclampsia; however, this relationship has been challenged by recent evidence that they may be separate disorders as preceding hypertension or proteinuria is absent in at least 15 to 20% of patients with HELLP syndrome.

Q2. What are diagnostic criteria of HELLP syndrome?

- *Primary diagnostic tools:*
    - Initial evaluation includes a thorough history, physical examination, blood pressure measurements, and blood and urine testing to detect the presence of proteinuria and /or end-organ involvement.
    - Obtain CBC with platelets, peripheral blood smear, and hepatic function panel (including AST, ALT, and bilirubin levels) and lactate dehydrogenase in patients with suspected preeclampsia or HELLP syndrome based on clinical presentation (typical symptoms, usually in association with hypertension and proteinuria).
    - Two methods of diagnosis are commonly used.
        1. *Tennessee classification:*
            - Hemolysis, indicated by 2 or more of the following: evidence of microangiopathic hemolysis on peripheral smear (schistocytes, burr cells); serum bilirubin 1.2 mg/dL or greater; serum haptoglobin 25 mg/dL or less or lactate dehydrogenase 2 or more times the upper level of normal; severe anemia not due to blood loss (hemoglobin 8–10 g/dL, depending on gestation)
            - Elevated liver enzymes, indicated by AST or ALT 2 or more times the upper level of normal.
            - Low platelets, indicated by platelet count less than 100,000/ mm^3.
            - HELLP is classified as complete when all 3 above findings are present and as partial or incomplete when just 1 or 2 is present.
        2. *American College of Obstetricians and Gynecologists criteria*:
            - Lactate dehydrogenase 600 IU/L or greater
            - AST and ALT 2 or more times the upper level of normal
            - Platelet count less than 100,000/mm^3
    - Obtain comprehensive metabolic panel, including creatinine concentration, disseminated intravascular coagulation panel, and urine protein concentration (24-hour urine collection or protein-creatinine ratio)
    - Assess fetal well-being with nonstress test and ultrasonographic evaluation to estimate fetal weight and amniotic fluid index; biophysical profile is indicated if nonstress test is nonreactive.
        - In potentially unstable situations, fetal monitoring is always performed first using bedside ultrasonography
    - Determine if the patient is in labor and evaluate the cervix with Bishop score.
- *Laboratory:*
    - *CBC:*
        - Platelet count less than 100,000/mm^3 is necessary to diagnose HELLP syndrome

- Platelet counts can decrease to as low as 6000/mm^3 (6×10^9/L), but any platelet count less than 150,000/mm^3 (150×10^9/L) warrants attention
- Mississippi subclassification assigns severity by nadir of thrombocytopenia but is not widely used clinically
- *Class I:* Platelet count less than 50,000/mm^3, AST or ALT 70 IU/L or higher, and lactate dehydrogenase 600 IU/L or higher
- *Class II:* Platelet count between 50,000/mm^3 and 100,000/mm^3, AST or ALT 70 IU/L or higher, and lactate dehydrogenase 600 IU/L or higher
- *Class III:* Platelet count between 100,000/mm^3 and 150,000/mm^3, AST or ALT 40 IU/L or higher, and lactate dehydrogenase 600 IU/L or higher
- Note that Class III levels do not meet commonly used diagnostic criteria

- Reticulocyte count can be increased.
- Hematocrit may be decreased or within the reference range and is typically the last of the abnormalities to appear; finding of decreased serum haptoglobin concentration may confirm ongoing hemolysis when hematocrit is within the reference range.

- *Peripheral blood smear:*
  - Microangiopathic hemolysis is suggested by presence of fragmented RBCs (schistocytes) or contracted, spiculated RBCs (Burr cells) in peripheral blood smear
- *Hepatic function panel:*
  - AST or ALT concentration of 70 units/L or higher is typical in HELLP syndrome:
    - Laboratory thresholds vary; diagnosis is based on AST and/or ALT more than 2 times the upper reference range for local laboratory.
  - Intravascular hemolysis is supported by elevated serum bilirubin concentration (at least 20.5 μmol/L or at least 1.2 mg/100 mL) and elevated lactate dehydrogenase concentration greater than 600 units/L (or at least 2 times the upper level of normal for laboratory range)
- *Serum haptoglobin level:*
  - Decrease is useful to corroborate the presence of intravascular hemolysis in conjunction with minimal microangiopathic changes in RBC morphology.
- *Urine protein to creatinine ratio:*
  - Proteinuria is defined by ratio 0.3 or greater (or protein of 300 mg or more in a 24-hour urine collection)

Review of the patient's condition and investigations is required in liaison with hematologists.

Q3. What are the risk factors for HELLP syndrome?

- *Age:*
  - The mean age of patients with HELLP syndrome is usually higher than the mean age of those with preeclampsia.
  - Persons aged 25 years or older are at higher risk for HELLP syndrome.
- *Genetics:*
  - HELLP syndrome demonstrates a familial tendency like preeclampsia; however, may have a different genetic basis than preeclampsia.
  - No single genetic cause has been identified; multiple gene variants along with environmental factors may contribute.
- *Ethnicity/race:*
  No clear evidence indicates persons of a particular race are at increased risk for HELLP syndrome:
  - However, higher rates of preeclampsia are seen in Black, Native American, and Alaskan Native patients
    - Among those with preeclampsia, higher rates of severe morbidity and mortality for both the patient and the fetus are seen among non-Hispanic Black patients than any other race or ethnicity
  - Differences in prevalence and outcomes appear to be linked to racial inequities, with mixed results in research on biological differences.
- *Other risk factors/associations:*
  - History of preeclampsia or HELLP syndrome
  - Unlike in preeclampsia, nulliparity is not a risk factor because at least 50% of patients with HELLP syndrome are multiparous.

Q4. What are the maternal and fetal complications?

- *Maternal complications:*
  Obstetric:
  - Eclampsia
  - Abruptio placentae
  - Wound hematoma or infection after cesarean delivery

  Coagulatory Disorders:
  - Disseminated intravascular coagulation
  - Recurrent thrombosis

  Neurological:
  - Cerebral edema
  - Cerebral hemorrhage
  - Retinal detachment
  - Cerebral infarction

Hepatic:
- Severe ascites
- Subcapsular liver hematoma
- Liver rupture
- Hepatic infarction

Renal:
- Acute renal failure

Respiratory:
- Pulmonary edema
- Acute respiratory distress syndrome
- Fetal complications:
- Intrauterine growth restriction
- Preterm delivery and associated complications
- Neonatal thrombocytopenia
- Respiratory distress syndrome

Q5. What is the differential diagnosis?

- *Pregnancy-related conditions:*
  - *Preeclampsia:*
    - Complication of pregnancy characterized by hypertension and proteinuria or, in the absence of proteinuria, by new onset of organ dysfunction
    - HELLP syndrome may represent a severe form of preeclampsia, and there is significant overlap in clinical and biochemical features
    - Like HELLP syndrome, preeclampsia may manifest with hypertension, proteinuria, epigastric pain, headache, and visual symptoms
    - Unlike HELLP syndrome, preeclampsia is more common in nulliparous females, and hypertension and proteinuria are always present
    - May be differentiated on basis of the following laboratory findings:
      - No evidence of microangiopathic hemolysis on peripheral blood smear
      - Platelet count may be within reference range (may be decreased in severe cases)
  - *Acute fatty liver of pregnancy:*
    - Rare complication of pregnancy caused by disordered maternal metabolism of fatty acids occurring in the third trimester
    - Clinical signs are variable, and in severe cases, there is significant overlap in clinical and biochemical features with HELLP syndrome
    - Like HELLP syndrome, acute fatty liver pregnancy typically occurs in the third trimester of pregnancy and manifests as

malaise, anorexia, nausea, vomiting, mid-epigastric or right upper abdominal pain, and headache

- Unlike most cases of HELLP syndrome, may be associated with jaundice and low-grade fever, and hypertension and proteinuria are usually absent
- May be differentiated based on the following laboratory findings:
  - Platelet count within reference range at presentation
  - Elevated WBC count, creatinine concentration, and bilirubin concentration
  - Prolonged prothrombin time or activated partial thromboplastin time
  - Antithrombin III activity reduced below 65%
  - Hypoglycemia

- *Nonpregnancy-related conditions:*
  - Conditions such as gastroenteritis, acute cholecystitis, appendicitis, and acute hepatitis may have similar clinical presentation with abdominal pain, malaise, nausea, and vomiting
    - Unlike HELLP, presenting symptoms are not associated with hypertension or proteinuria
    - Differentiated on the basis of history, clinical features, and laboratory findings:
      - No evidence of microangiopathic hemolysis on peripheral blood smear; platelet count within reference range
  - Thrombotic thrombocytopenic purpura and hemolytic uremic syndrome also have hemolysis, and thrombocytopenia, and may have similar clinical presentation (e.g., nausea, vomiting, abdominal pain, headache)
    - Unlike HELLP, the elevation of AST and ALT is usually mild and anemia is more prominent

Q6. What is management of HELLP?

Treatment options: Promptly initiate antihypertensive therapy in patients who have persistent (15 minutes or more) hypertension with systolic blood pressure higher than 160 mm Hg or diastolic blood pressure higher than 110 mm Hg, or both.

- The optimal target has not been determined, but protocols recommend systolic blood pressure lower than 160 mm Hg and diastolic blood pressure lower than 100 mm Hg.
- Lowering blood pressure too much may be harmful; avoid systolic blood pressure lower than 120 mm Hg or diastolic blood pressure lower than 80 mm Hg. If the patient is already established on daily antihypertensive therapy, choose an agent from a different drug class of current regimen.

- For treatment during pregnancy, use fetal surveillance during anti-hypertensive treatment if the fetus is viable.
  Administer magnesium sulfate for seizure prophylaxis.
  Delivery is the definitive treatment for cases during pregnancy (although postpartum cases occur):
  - Timing of delivery depends on gestational age and conditions of the patient and fetus:
    - Deliver immediately after patient stabilization in the following:
      - Pregnancies at 34 weeks of gestation or longer
      - Pregnancies shorter than 23 weeks of gestation or if fetus is nonviable
      - Pregnancies between 23 and 34 weeks of gestation if there is disseminated intravascular coagulation, liver infarction or hemorrhage, renal failure, pulmonary edema, suspected abruptio placentae, or nonreassuring fetal status
      - Administering corticosteroids for fetal lung maturation is recommended, but do not delay delivery to complete course
  - Deliver within 24–48 hours after patient stabilization in pregnancies between 23 and 34 weeks of gestation, provided patient and fetus remain stable
  - Administering corticosteroids for fetal lung maturation is recommended, but do not complete course if condition of pregnant patient or fetus deteriorates
- Route of delivery is selected on the condition of patient, the basis of gestational age, fetal presentation, cervical status, obstetric history, and fetal condition.
  - Cesarean delivery is recommended for standard obstetric indications (e.g., unfavorable cervix, oligohydramnios) and where an emergent delivery is required.
  - Platelet transfusion before vaginal delivery is recommended by if platelet count is less than 20,000/mm^3 and before cesarean delivery if less than 50,000/mm^3; the precise threshold is determined in consultation with the hematologist.
  - Spinal or epidural anesthesia is recommended if analgesia or anesthesia is required for delivery
    - No definitive lower limit platelet count is known for neuraxial anesthesia; however, the risk of epidural hematoma is exceptionally low in patients with stable platelet counts 70,000/mm^3 without anticoagulants or coagulopathy
- Expectant management is not typically recommended.
  - Expectant management before completing 34 weeks of gestation may be an acceptable option in carefully selected patients if it is performed

in tertiary care units under close surveillance; however, there is limited evidence that this is beneficial. Not recommended if neonate is not expected to survive

- Deliver immediately if fetal or maternal condition deteriorates during expectant management

- Corticosteroids do not appear to reduce mortality and morbidity (more evidence needed)

May improve maternal platelet counts (more evidence needed)

- May be considered in settings in which improved platelet count is clinically important.

Drug therapy:

- *Antihypertensive drugs:*
    - *Labetalol:*
        - *Bolus dose:*
            - *Labetalol:* Hydrochloride solution for injection; Adults: 10–20 mg IV, then 20–80 mg IV every 10–30 minutes until goal blood pressure is attained. Maximum cumulative dose: 300 mg
        - *Continuous infusion:*
            - *Labetalol:* Hydrochloride solution for injection; Adults: 0.5–2 mg/minute continuous IV infusion, initially. Titrate dose every 15 minutes until goal blood pressure is attained. Maximum: 10 mg/minute. Maximum cumulative dose: 300 mg.
    - *Calcium channel blocker:*
        - *Nifedipine (immediate release):*
            - *Nifedipine oral capsule; adults:* 10–20 mg PO every 15–30 minutes, then 10–20 mg PO every 2–6 hours until blood pressure control is attained. Maximum: 180 mg/day
    - *Vasodilator:*
        - *Hydralazine (caution vigilant management):*
            - *Bolus dose:*

              Hydralazine: Hydrochloride solution for injection; adults: 5 mg IV, then 5–10 mg IV every 20–40 minutes until goal blood pressure is attained. Maximum cumulative dose: 20 mg.
        - *Continuous infusion:*
            - *Hydralazine:* Hydrochloride solution for injection; adults: 0.5–5 mg/hour continuous IV infusion, initially. Titrate by 1–2 mg/h every 15–20 minutes until goal blood pressure is attained. Maximum: 10 mg/h.
    - In case of teenage pregnancy, appropriate dose needs to be calculated.

- *Antenatal corticosteroids:*
  - *Betamethasone:*
    - Betamethasone acetate, betamethasone sodium phosphate suspension for injection; Adults: 12 mg IM every 24 hours for 2 doses. Consider a repeat or rescue course when at risk of preterm delivery within the next 7 days and prior course administered more than 14 days previously. Rescue course could be provided as early as 7 days from the prior dose if indicated by clinical situation.
- *Seizure prophylaxis:*
  - *Magnesium sulfate:*
    - *Intravenous (recommended):* Magnesium sulfate solution for injection; Adults: 4–6 g IV loading dose, followed by 1–2 g/hour continuous IV infusion for at least 24 hours. Maximum: 30–40 g/24 hours.
    - *Intramuscular (if platelet count is above 750,000):* Magnesium sulfate solution for injection; Adults: 10 g IM loading dose, followed by 5 g IM every 4 hours for at least 24 hours. Maximum: 30–40 g/24 hours.

Nondrug and supportive care:

- Administer IV fluids
- Closely monitor vital signs and fluid balance
- Consider platelet transfusion in actively bleeding patients with platelet count less than 50,000/mm^3, before vaginal delivery in those with platelet count less than 20,000/mm^3, and before cesarean delivery in those with platelet count less than 40,000 to 50,000/mm^3.
- Because evidence is limited regarding indications for platelet transfusion, consult hematology and anesthesiology specialists to determine thresholds.

Q7. What is postpartum HELLP syndrome and recurrence in future pregnancy?

- HELLP that develops after delivery
- Most within 48 hours but can occur up to 7 days after delivery
- Risk of renal failure and pulmonary edema is significantly higher than with pre-partum HELLP
- For persistent hemolysis, thrombocytopenia, and hypoproteinemia, RBC and platelet transfusion and protein supplementation are standard therapy
- Patients with HELLP syndrome might have an increased risk of future cardiovascular and metabolic disease (e.g., hypertension, elevated BMI, elevated glucose, metabolic syndrome, unfavorable lipid parameters)

based on studies of patients with preeclampsia and eclampsia, some of which included those with HELLP syndrome

- Counseling of lifestyle diseases like hypertension, obesity, and other comorbid conditions is essential.
- Fetal prognosis is strongly influenced by the gestational age at delivery; prognosis is poorer with delivery at earlier gestational ages. Perinatal death was reported in 7.4% to 34% of patients.
- Patients with HELLP syndrome have a 19% to 27% risk of developing HELLP syndrome in subsequent pregnancies.
- Recurrent cases occur in the latter part of the gestation period and are less severe after two episodes.
- No specific screening tests; early antenatal care and more frequent antenatal monitoring are required.
- There is no specific preventive therapy for HELLP syndrome; however, daily low-dose aspirin after 12 weeks of gestation is recommended to reduce risk of preeclampsia in those at high risk.
- Contraceptive advice at the time of discharge for these patients is necessary. Barrier, LARC methods can be used. Low-dose oral contraceptives are safe in women with prior HELLP.

12.4 DISSEMINATED INTRAVASCULAR COAGULATION

T Ramanidevi

Q1. What is the prevalence of DIC in obstetrics?

Disseminated intravascular coagulation (DIC) is a serious condition that can occur in obstetrics, often associated with severe complications. DIC is an acquired syndrome characterized by the intravascular activation of the coagulation cascade. The prevalence of DIC in obstetric patients varies, but certain conditions significantly increase the risk. Prevalence of DIC in obstetric is 0.03 to 0.35%. Early recognition and management are crucial to improving outcomes for both the mother and the baby.

Q2. What are the reasons for DIC in obstetrics?

1. *Placental abruption:* This condition has a strong association with DIC, with studies indicating that up to 30% of cases can develop DIC.
2. *Amniotic fluid embolism:* Rare but highly fatal, DIC is present in a significant percentage of these cases.
3. *Sepsis:* Obstetric sepsis can lead to DIC in a notable proportion of affected individuals.
4. *Preeclampsia/eclampsia:* Severe cases can sometimes progress to DIC.
5. *Intrauterine fetal demise:* Prolonged retention of a deceased fetus can lead to DIC.

6. Massive hemorrhage
7. Acute fatty liver
8. Amniotic fluid embolism.

Overall, the incidence of DIC in obstetrics is relatively low but becomes significant in the presence of these high-risk conditions.

Q3. What are the types of DIC?

Disseminated intravascular coagulation (DIC) can be classified into two main types based on the onset and progression of symptoms—acute and chronic.

It can also be classified as subclinical, procoagulant, or hyperfibrinolytic DIC, based on which pathway is predominantly activated.

- *Subclinical:* Balanced coagulation and fibrinolytic pathways.
- *Procoagulant DIC:* Pre-dominance of coagulation pathway activation
- *Hyperfibrinolytic DIC:* Predominance of fibrinolytic pathway activation

1. *Acute DIC:*
    - *Characteristics:* Rapid onset and progression, often presenting with severe bleeding and clotting issues simultaneously.
    - *Causes:* Commonly associated with severe trauma, obstetric emergencies (such as placental abruption or amniotic fluid embolism), sepsis, and major surgery.
    - *Clinical features:* Patients may exhibit widespread hemorrhage, petechiae, ecchymoses, and oozing from venipuncture sites. Laboratory findings typically show low platelet counts, prolonged clotting times, and elevated levels of fibrin degradation products (D-dimers).
2. *Chronic DIC*:
    - *Characteristics:* Gradual onset with milder, more prolonged symptoms. Thrombosis may be more prominent than bleeding.
    - *Causes:* Often associated with chronic conditions such as cancer (especially mucin-producing adenocarcinomas), chronic liver disease, and vascular abnormalities.
    - *Clinical features:* Patients may present with thrombotic complications such as deep vein thrombosis or pulmonary embolism. Laboratory findings may show milder abnormalities in coagulation tests compared to acute DIC, with some patients exhibiting normal platelet counts and clotting time.

Both types require prompt medical attention, but their management strategies can differ based on the underlying cause and the severity of the condition.

Q4. What are the triggers that lead to DIC?

Disseminated intravascular coagulation (DIC) can be triggered by a variety of underlying conditions and events that lead to widespread activation of the clotting cascade. Here are some common triggers:

1. *Infections:*
   - *Sepsis:* Particularly from gram-negative bacteria, but also from gram-positive bacteria, viruses, fungi, and parasites.
2. *Obstetric complications*:
   - Placental abruption
   - Amniotic fluid embolism
   - Severe preeclampsia/eclampsia
   - Retained dead fetus
3. *Malignancies:*
   - Acute promyelocytic leukemia (APL)
   - Mucin-producing adenocarcinomas
4. *Severe trauma*:
   - *Massive tissue injury:* From accidents, burns, or major surgery.
5. *Vascular abnormalities:*
   - *Aortic aneurysm:* Abnormal dilation of the aorta
   - *Giant hemangiomas:* Benign tumors of blood vessels (Kasabach-Merritt syndrome)
6. *Liver disease:*
   - *Acute liver failure:* Leading to impaired synthesis of clotting factors
   - *Chronic liver disease:* Resulting in coagulopathy and increased risk of DIC
7. *Transfusion reactions:*
   - *Hemolytic transfusion reactions:* Due to incompatible blood transfusion
8. *Immunologic disorders:*
   - *Systemic lupus erythematosus (SLE):* An autoimmune disease that can lead to DIC in severe cases.
9. *Severe inflammatory conditions:*
   - Pancreatitis
   - Heat stroke

   Each of these triggers can initiate a complex cascade of events leading to the widespread formation of clots within the blood vessels, consumption of clotting factors and platelets, and a subsequent risk of severe bleeding. The underlying condition must be identified and managed alongside supportive care for DIC.

Q5. What is diagnosis of DIC, clinical definition, and laboratory findings?

The diagnosis of disseminated intravascular coagulation (DIC) is based on clinical presentation and laboratory findings. No single test can diagnose DIC, so a combination of clinical criteria and laboratory tests are used.

Clinical definition: DIC is characterized by systemic activation of blood coagulation, leading to the generation and deposition of fibrin, resulting in microvascular thrombi in various organs, contributing to organ dysfunction. Simultaneously, the consumption of platelets and coagulation factors leads to bleeding.

Laboratory findings:

1. *Platelet count:* Typically decreased (thrombocytopenia) due to consumption of platelets in clot formation.
2. *Coagulation tests:*
   - *Prothrombin time (PT):* Prolonged.
   - *Activated partial thromboplastin time (aPTT):* Prolonged.
3. *Fibrinogen level:* Decreased, as it is consumed during widespread clotting.
4. *D-dimer:* Elevated, reflecting increased fibrinolysis and breakdown of fibrin clots.
5. *Fibrin degradation products (FDPs):* Elevated, indicating enhanced fibrinolysis.
6. *Peripheral blood smear:* Presence of schistocytes (fragmented red blood cells) due to mechanical damage in microcirculation.

Scoring systems:

To aid in the diagnosis of DIC, several scoring systems have been developed, such as the International Society on Thrombosis and Haemostasis (ISTH) DIC score. The ISTH score considers the following parameters:

- Platelet count
- PT prolongation
- Fibrinogen level
- D-dimer or FDP levels

Examples of ISTH DIC scoring:

- Platelet count (>100 x 10^9/L = 0, <100 x 10^9/L = 1, <50 x 10^9/L = 2)
- PT prolongation (<3 seconds = 0, 3–6 seconds = 1, >6 seconds = 2)
- Fibrinogen level (>1 g/L = 0, <1 g/L = 1)
- D-dimer or FDPs (no increase = 0, moderate increase = 2, strong increase = 3)
- A score of 5 or more is suggestive of DIC.

Clinical features:

- *Bleeding:* From venipuncture sites, mucous membranes, gastrointestinal tract, or other sites.

- *Thrombosis:* Manifestations depend on the location of clots, which may include organ dysfunction such as renal failure, liver dysfunction, respiratory distress, or neurological symptoms.
- *Organ dysfunction:* Due to microvascular thrombosis and hemorrhage.

Q6. What are some of the experimental therapies for DIC?

Experimental therapies for disseminated intravascular coagulation (DIC) are focused on managing the underlying condition, supporting coagulation, and mitigating the effects of excessive clotting and bleeding. Here are some experimental and emerging therapies:

Anticoagulants like recombinant thrombomodulin, direct thrombin inhibitors (e.g., argatroban, dabigatran), direct factor Xa Inhibitors (e.g., rivaroxaban, apixaban), anti-inflammatory agents, antithrombin III concentrates, activated protein C (e.g., drotrecogin alfa), hemostatic agents like fibrinogen concentrates, and prothrombin complex concentrates (PCCs) are under evaluation.

Drugs modulating coagulation and inflammation like tissue factor pathway inhibitors, anti-inflammatory cytokine therapies, gene therapy and novel biologicals agents are under trial.

Supportive and adjunctive therapies like extracorporeal blood purification and stem cell therapies under research setting are showing promising results.

While these experimental therapies show promise, they are often in the investigational or early clinical trial phases. Standard treatment for DIC still relies heavily on addressing the underlying cause, supportive care, and careful management of coagulation and bleeding.

Q7. What is a massive transfusion protocol?

A massive transfusion protocol (MTP) is a standardized approach used in medical settings to manage patients who require rapid and large-volume blood transfusions, typically due to severe hemorrhage. The goal of an MTP is to ensure the timely and balanced administration of blood products to prevent coagulopathy, hypothermia, acidosis, and to stabilize the patient.

Here are the key components and principles of an MTP. One indication for MTP is obstetric hemorrhage where the loss of more than 30% of blood volume (approximately 1.5 liters in adults), need for transfusion of 10 or more units of packed red blood cells (PRBCs) within 24 hours and transfusion of more than 4 units of PRBCs in one hour with ongoing bleeding. Components of MTP: Packed Red Blood Cells (PRBCs), Fresh Frozen Plasma (FFP), Platelets and Cryoprecipitate. A common ratio is 1:1:1 or 1:1:2 of PRBCs: FFP: Platelets to prevent dilutional coagulopathy. Adjunctive Therapies like Tranexamic Acid, Calcium Gluconate or Calcium Chloride to address hypocalcemia due to citrate in blood products. Continuous monitoring of vital signs, including blood pressure, heart rate, and oxygen saturation and regular assessment of laboratory values such as hemoglobin, hematocrit, coagulation parameters (PT, aPTT, fibrinogen), and electrolytes. Monitoring for signs of coagulopathy, acidosis, and hypothermia are very important. Efficient communication and coordination among the medical team, blood bank, and other departments are essential. Massive Transfusion Protocol is a critical, lifesaving intervention for managing severe hemorrhage. It involves the coordinated delivery of blood products and adjunctive therapies in a standardized manner to restore hemostasis, correct coagulopathy, and stabilize the patient.

Q8. Why do you prefer component therapy to whole blood transfusion?

Blood component therapy is often preferred over whole blood transfusion for several reasons, including the ability to target specific deficiencies, reduce risks, and optimize the use of blood resources. Here are the key reasons for preferring blood component therapy.

Targeted therapy:

1. *Specific treatment of deficiencies:* Packed red blood cells (PRBCs) are used to treat anemia and improve oxygen-carrying capacity.
2. Fresh frozen plasma (FFP) provides clotting factors for patients with coagulopathies.
3. Platelets are used to treat or prevent bleeding in patients with thrombocytopenia or platelet dysfunction.
4. Cryoprecipitate provides fibrinogen and other specific clotting factors for patients with deficiencies. Tailored therapy allows clinicians to administer only the components needed, reducing the risk of volume overload and other complications associated with whole blood transfusion.

There are reduced risks of transfusion reactions, lower the risk of allergic reactions, febrile reactions, and other transfusion-related complications by limiting exposure to unnecessary components. This decreases the risk of transfusion-associated circulatory overload (TACO), lowers the risk of transfusion-related acute lung injury (TRALI). A single unit of donated whole blood can be separated into multiple components (PRBCs, plasma, platelets), allowing treatment of several patients from one donation. Blood banks can better manage supplies and meet specific demands for different components, ensuring availability for patients in need.

Therapeutic advantages are it can minimize the risk of complications and avoid the administration of unnecessary cells or proteins. Some components can be leukocyte-reduced, irradiated, or pathogen-reduced to further enhance safety for immunocompromised patients or those with specific conditions.

In summary blood component therapy offers significant advantages over whole blood transfusion by allowing targeted treatment of specific deficiencies, reducing the risk of complications, optimizing the use of donated blood, and improving overall patient care. These benefits make blood component therapy the standard practice in modern transfusion medicine.

Q9. What is the prothrombin complex concentrate?

Prothrombin complex concentrate (PCC) is a medication used to treat and prevent bleeding in patients with deficiencies in clotting factors. PCC is a concentrated mixture of several blood clotting factors, which are usually extracted from donated human plasma. These concentrates typically include: Factor II (Prothrombin), Factor VII, Factor IX and Factor X. Some formulations may also contain proteins C and S, which are natural anticoagulants. PCC is primarily used massive transfusion, or disseminated intravascular coagulation (DIC). It can lead to thromboembolic events.

Q10. What is plateletpheresis?

Plateletpheresis is a process by which platelets are collected from one single donor. The harvested platelets from 1 unit will be equal to 6 units of random donor platelets.

Q11. What is the difference between single donor platelet and random donor platelets?

Single donor platelet is leukoreduced and hence reduced risk of sepsis and transfusion reaction. Random donor platelets are taken from multiple donors. Random donor platelets amounting to 6 units are equivalent to 1 unit of SDP, but has more WBCs which require filtration and therefore has increased risk of complications.

Q12. What is the lethal triad in coagulopathy?

Lethal triad also known as triad of death are hypothermia, acidosis, and coagulopathy.

Hypothermia below 35°C impairs function of enzymes involved in coagulation, reduces platelet function and aggravates DIC. It can also lead to myocardial infarction and arrhythmias.

Acidosis is defined as a pH below 7.35. This may be due to blood loss leading to anaerobic metabolism and lactic acid production. Use of resuscitation fluid and blood products can contribute to acidosis which can impair clotting factors and enzymes which exacerbates coagulopathy, cardiovascular instability and cardiac dysfunction.

Coagulopathy results in continuous bleeding which further leads to hypothermia and acidosis. Hence prevention of hypothermia, correction of acidosis and massive transfusion protocol to be followed to correct coagulopathy. Hypocalcemia needs to be corrected. Basic pathology to be corrected.

Q13. What is the most useful point of care test in the management of DIC?

Thromboelastography, it is graphic representation of the clotting process done in the TEG-ROTEM analyzer. The test guides the care giver on what component needs to be transfused in the management of massive obstetric hemorrhage.

Q14. Does DIC recur in subsequent pregnancies?

It can recur in pregnancy up to 50%, when associated with protein S deficiency; in pregnancy associated TTP and atypical hemolytic uremic syndrome, it is 10–30%; following placental abruption it is 5.8%. Proper monitoring, prophylaxis, and early treatment are crucial.

Q15. Does DIC amount to severe acute maternal morbidity?

Yes, DIC is considered a severe acute maternal morbidity. It is associated with high levels of maternal morbidity and mortality, contributing to up to 25% of maternal deaths. Conditions leading to DIC, such as placental abruption and severe hemorrhage, often result in significant complications like massive transfusions, hysterectomy, and intensive care unit admissions.

Q16. What is the role factor VIIa in DIC?

Factor VIIa (recombinant activated factor VII) plays a significant but specialized role in the management of Disseminated Intravascular Coagulation (DIC). DIC is a complex condition characterized by widespread activation of the coagulation cascade, leading to both thrombotic and bleeding complications due to the consumption of clotting factors and platelets. The use of factor VIIa in DIC is controversial and should be approached with caution.

Factor VIIa primarily acts to enhance hemostasis by activating the extrinsic pathway of coagulation, which leads to the formation of a clot. In severe cases of DIC, especially when patients have uncontrolled bleeding despite conventional measures (e.g., fresh frozen plasma, platelet transfusions), factor VIIa has been used as a rescue therapy to achieve hemostasis. Since DIC often involves a delicate balance between clotting and bleeding, the use of factor VIIa is typically reserved for cases of life-threatening hemorrhage where standard therapies have failed. It can promote clot formation in areas of tissue injury, helping to stabilize bleeding. A major concern with factor VIIa is the risk of inducing or exacerbating thromboembolic events, which are already a complication of DIC due to widespread activation of clotting factors. Thus, it is used with extreme caution, particularly in patients who may have a higher risk of thrombotic events (e.g., those with underlying cardiovascular disease). It serves as a temporary hemostatic agent while efforts to address the root cause of DIC continue. Without resolving the underlying cause, the benefit of using factor VIIa may be short-lived. The evidence for the efficacy of recombinant factor VIIa in DIC management is limited. Most recommendations are based on case reports and small studies. It does not correct the underlying cause for DIC. Due to the high cost and potential risks, its use remains off-label and is considered on a case-by-case basis in critically ill patients.

12.5 PREECLAMPSIA AND PULMONARY EDEMA

Prakash K Mehta

INTRODUCTION

Pulmonary edema in pregnant women is an uncommon but life-threatening event with high maternal and perinatal morbidity and mortality. It is a state of abnormal fluid accumulation in the alveolar space of the lung and can interfere with normal oxygenation and ventilation.

Pulmonary edema is the main cardiovascular complication of preeclampsia and one of the criteria of severe preeclampsia; occurs in 3% of preeclampsia cases, 70% of which take place during postpartum. It is defined as the sudden onset of breathlessness and accompanying symptoms including orthopnea, agitation, and cough, associated with clinical signs of tachycardia, tachypnea, crepitations and rhonchi, gallop rhythm, murmurs on cardiac auscultation and decreased oxygen saturation. Prompt diagnosis and management are very important for the survival of the patient. Considerations should include physiological changes of pregnancy, the risk of aspiration and difficult airway, reduced respiratory and metabolic reserve, avoidance of aortocaval compression, and delivery of the fetus. Immediate management of acute pulmonary edema includes oxygenation, ventilation, and circulation control with vasodilators.

Q1. Why and when does pulmonary edema occur in patients with preeclampsia?

Pulmonary edema should be ruled out in case of dyspnea in a pregnant woman.

Normally, the heart, lungs, and vascular system work in concert to facilitate fluid movement through the capillary and lymphatics of the lung and ensure adequate oxygenation, with limited transudation of fluid from the lung tissue into the alveolar space. In disease states causing acute lung injury (ALI), both direct and indirect, this harmony is disrupted.

Timing of development:

Antepartum: Pulmonary edema is less common before delivery, but can develop during pregnancy in severe cases of preeclampsia, particularly as blood pressure rises and fluid balance becomes more precarious.

Intrapartum: Pulmonary edema during labor is rare but can occur due to the stress and strain on the cardiovascular system during contractions and pushing.

Postpartum: This is the most common period for the development of pulmonary edema in preeclampsia. It typically occurs within the first 48 hours after delivery but can manifest up to a week postpartum. The sudden removal of the placenta leads to changes in vascular tone and volume status, which can exacerbate fluid shifts and predispose to pulmonary edema.

Q2. What pathophysiological changes in cases of preeclampsia make the woman more prone to pulmonary edema?

Pregnancy is associated with physiological adaptations, making these women more prone to developing pulmonary edema. Both pulmonary vascular resistance and systemic vascular resistance, decrease significantly in normal pregnancy. The colloid osmotic pressure/pulmonary capillary wedge pressure gradient is reduced by about 30%, making pregnant women particularly susceptible to pulmonary edema. Pulmonary edema will be precipitated if there is either an increase in cardiac preload (such as infusion of fluids) increased pulmonary capillary permeability (such as in preeclampsia) or both.

Pathophysiology: Many mechanisms have been proposed to explain the pathogenesis of pulmonary edema in severe preeclampsia including hypervolemia, left ventricular failure, and pulmonary capillary leakage. However, it is thought that increased systemic vascular resistance induces significant changes in loading conditions of the ventricular myocardium contributing to diastolic filling abnormalities and the development of an ischemic substrate with the potential for development of heart failure, pulmonary edema, and/or sudden death. The movement of fluid is dependent on Starling's law and influenced by both hydrostatic and oncotic pressures.

In summary, the pathophysiology of pulmonary edema in preeclampsia involves a combination of endothelial dysfunction, increased capillary permeability, hemodynamic changes, inflammatory responses, fluid retention, cardiac dysfunction, renal abnormalities, and coagulation disturbances. Pulmonary edema will occur if there is an increase in cardiac preload (such as infusion of fluids), increased pulmonary capillary permeability (such as in preeclampsia), or both. Although both blood volume and stroke volume increase in pregnancy, pulmonary capillary wedge pressure and central venous pressure do not increase significantly. Pulmonary vascular resistance (PVR), like systemic vascular resistance (SVR), decreases significantly in normal pregnancy. Although the pulmonary capillary wedge pressure (PCWP) does not alter, serum colloid osmotic pressure is decreased by 10–15%. The colloid osmotic pressure/pulmonary capillary wedge pressure gradient is reduced by about 30%, making pregnant women particularly susceptible to pulmonary edema. Pulmonary edema will be precipitated if there is either an increase in cardiac preload (such as infusion of fluids) increased pulmonary capillary permeability (such as in preeclampsia) or both. Labor is associated with further increases in cardiac output (15% in the first stage and 50% in the second stage). Uterine contractions lead to an autotransfusion of 300–500 mL of blood back into the circulation. Added to this is a sympathetic response to pain and anxiety, which further elevates the heart rate and blood pressure. Following delivery, there is an immediate rise in cardiac output due to relief of the inferior vena cava obstruction and contraction of the uterus, which empties blood into the systemic circulation. Cardiac output increases by 60–80%, followed by a rapid decline in prelabor values within about one hour of delivery. The fluid shift from extravascular space increases the venous return and stroke volume further.

Q3. What are the risk factors for pulmonary edema?

Factors contributing to incidence:

1. *Severe hypertension:* Poorly controlled hypertension is a significant risk factor. Elevated blood pressure associated with preeclampsia can strain the heart and pulmonary vasculature, contributing to fluid leakage into the lungs.
2. *Endothelial dysfunction:* Preeclampsia is characterized by widespread endothelial dysfunction, which affects the lining of blood vessels throughout the body, including those in the lungs. Endothelial dysfunction leads to increased vascular permeability, allowing fluid and proteins to leak out of the blood vessels and into the surrounding tissues.
3. *Fluid retention and increased blood volume:* Preeclampsia can cause fluid retention throughout the body, leading to an increase in blood volume. This can overload the heart's capacity to pump effectively.
4. *Fluid overload:* Aggressive fluid administration, especially during labor or after delivery, can exacerbate fluid shifts. Administration of too much intravenous (IV) fluid and transfusion of blood products have been described as causal factors in many studies.
5. *Capillary leak syndrome:* Preeclampsia may induce a systemic inflammatory response and endothelial dysfunction, which can lead

to increased permeability of capillaries. This increased permeability allows fluid to leak out of the blood vessels and into the surrounding tissues, including the lungs.

6. *Activation of inflammatory pathways:* Preeclampsia involves an inflammatory response characterized by the release of cytokines and other inflammatory mediators. These substances contribute to endothelial activation and further increase vascular permeability, exacerbating fluid leakage into the lungs.
7. *Renal dysfunction:* Impaired kidney function can lead to fluid retention and imbalance. The contribution of renal dysfunction to the formation of pulmonary edema has been attributed to bulk fluid accumulation, which increases capillary hydrostatic pressure, and creates a gradient favoring net flow of fluid into the alveolar spaces. The crosstalk between the kidney and the lung in the critically ill patient is of extreme importance.
8. *Cardiac dysfunction:* Pre-existing or pregnancy-induced cardiac issues increase the risk. Preeclampsia can sometimes cause heart dysfunction, such as left ventricular diastolic dysfunction, which impairs the heart's ability to relax and fill properly. This can lead to congestion in the lungs and the development of pulmonary edema.
9. *Coagulation abnormalities:* Preeclampsia is associated with abnormalities in coagulation factors and fibrinolysis. These changes can lead to microthrombi formation and microvascular occlusion, further impairing pulmonary circulation and contributing to pulmonary edema.
10. *Multigravidity and age:* Higher parity and extremes of maternal age may also contribute.
11. *Frequently used medications:* Possibly associated with the development of pulmonary edema were $MgSO_4$ and oxytocin. Yet, these medications are also potentially life-saving as part of the management of preeclampsia and often used to induce labor and prevent postpartum hemorrhage. Close monitoring of already sick women is needed when these drugs are administered.

Managing these risk factors through careful monitoring of blood pressure, fluid balance, and kidney function is crucial in preventing pulmonary edema in women with preeclampsia.

Q4. When to suspect that a preeclampsia patient has developed pulmonary edema?

Recognizing pulmonary edema in a patient with preeclampsia is critical for prompt management and intervention. Signs and symptoms that should raise suspicion of pulmonary edema in a patient with preeclampsia include:

1. *Respiratory symptoms:*
   - Sudden onset or worsening of shortness of breath (dyspnea)
   - Orthopnea (difficulty breathing while lying flat)
   - Paroxysmal nocturnal dyspnea (sudden onset of difficulty breathing at night)
   - Rapid breathing (tachypnea)
2. *Cardiovascular symptoms:*
   - Chest pain or discomfort
   - Palpitations or irregular heartbeat
   - Cold, clammy skin
3. *General signs:*
   - Sudden weight gain or swelling (edema) not explained by other factors
   - Cough, especially if it is productive of frothy or pink-tinged sputum
4. *Clinical findings:*
   - Crackles or rales are heard on auscultation of the lungs
   - Elevated jugular venous pressure (JVP) indicating fluid overload
   - Signs of respiratory distress such as use of accessory muscles
5. *Laboratory and diagnostic tests:*
   - Chest X-ray may show characteristic findings such as diffuse bilateral infiltrates ("bat wing" appearance).
   - Arterial blood gas analysis may reveal respiratory alkalosis or hypoxemia.
   - Elevated brain natriuretic peptide (BNP) levels, although these are not routinely measured in all settings.
6. *Clinical context:*
   - Rapid deterioration in clinical status despite adequate treatment for hypertension and other preeclampsia symptoms.
   - Development of new or worsening hypertension and proteinuria along with respiratory symptoms should also raise suspicion.

Q5. What are the clinical findings, investigations, and imaging studies?

Preeclampsia is associated with many clinical symptoms (breathlessness, orthopnea, agitation, and cough) and signs (tachycardia, tachypnea, crackles and wheeze on chest auscultation, S3 gallop rhythm and murmurs, decreased oxygen saturation). Typical chest X-ray features include upper lobe redistribution, Kerley-B lines, and pulmonary infiltrates.

Clinical presentation:

- Patients may present with worsening shortness of breath, cough, frothy sputum, and sometimes chest pain.
- Crackles (rales) may be heard on auscultation of the lungs, indicating fluid accumulation in the alveoli.

- Oxygen saturation may be decreased, and the patient may appear anxious or cyanotic.

  Attention to the incidence of PPCM in patients with acute PE is equally important.

Investigations:
- Complete blood count
- Blood chemistry
- Pulse oximetry
- Arterial blood gases
- Chest X-ray and Chest CT scan
- Echocardiography and ECG
- Point of care test like IVC collapsibility to assess fluid status.

Q6. How to proceed with treatment once the diagnosis is confirmed?

If pulmonary edema is suspected, immediate medical evaluation and intervention are necessary. Prompt management typically involves ensuring adequate oxygenation, diuresis to reduce fluid overload, and careful monitoring of cardiovascular status. Close monitoring of both maternal and fetal status is crucial in managing this condition effectively. It is essential to involve obstetric and medical teams promptly to ensure comprehensive care and to prevent further deterioration.

1. *Supportive care:* Oxygen therapy to improve oxygenation and reduce respiratory distress.
2. *Monitoring and supportive measures:*
   a. *Hemodynamic monitoring:* Close monitoring of blood pressure, heart rate, and cardiac output is crucial to manage fluid status and optimize cardiac function.
   b. *Fluid management:* Careful fluid management is essential to avoid exacerbating pulmonary edema. Diuretics may be used to reduce fluid overload under close monitoring of urine output and electrolyte balance.
3. *Positioning:*
   Semi-Fowler's position: Elevating the head of the bed to 30–45° helps to improve lung mechanics and reduce venous return to the heart, thereby decreasing pulmonary congestion.
4. *Treatment of underlying cause:* Addressing the underlying cause of pulmonary edema is essential. In the context of preeclampsia, delivery of the baby and placenta often resolves the condition.
5. *Diuretics:* Diuretics play a critical role in managing pulmonary edema, including that which may occur in conditions like severe preeclampsia. They are used to reduce fluid overload and alleviate pulmonary congestion. By promoting the excretion of sodium and water via the kidneys, diuretics

alleviate pulmonary congestion and improve respiratory symptoms such as dyspnea and oxygenation. Loop diuretics like Furosemide are particularly effective in managing acute pulmonary edema due to their potent diuretic action and rapid onset of action.

Initial dose: For acute pulmonary edema, an initial intravenous dose of 20–40 mg of furosemide is often given.

Titration: Dosing may be titrated based on response, with repeated doses every 20–30 minutes if necessary, up to a maximum dose of 160–200 mg/day.

Close monitoring of urine output, electrolytes (especially potassium), and renal function is essential during diuretic therapy.

6. *Blood pressure control:* Antihypertensive medications may be used cautiously to manage blood pressure.
7. *Delivery of the baby:* Definitive treatment often involves delivery of the baby and placenta, as the underlying cause of preeclampsia cannot be resolved until pregnancy is terminated.
8. *Ventilation in pulmonary edema:* Ventilation strategies in the management of pulmonary edema aim to improve oxygenation and reduce the work of breathing while addressing the underlying cause of fluid accumulation in the lungs.
   a. *Oxygen therapy*:

      Supplemental oxygen: Administering high-flow oxygen through a mask or nasal cannula is typically the initial step to improve oxygenation and relieve hypoxemia.

      Oxygen saturation monitoring: Continuous monitoring of oxygen saturation helps guide the adequacy of oxygen therapy.

      Noninvasive ventilation (NIV): NIV is indicated for patients with moderate to severe respiratory distress who can protect their airway and maintain respiratory drive.

      Continuous positive airway pressure (CPAP) or bi-level positive airway pressure (BiPAP): NIV can be beneficial in pulmonary edema by providing positive pressure to keep alveoli open during expiration and reducing the work of breathing. It also helps to decrease preload on the heart and improve gas exchange.

      Invasive mechanical ventilation:

      Endotracheal intubation: Patients who do not improve with NIV or who have severe respiratory failure may require intubation and mechanical ventilation.

      Positive pressure ventilation: Mechanical ventilation aims to optimize oxygenation and ventilation parameters, including tidal volume, respiratory rate, and positive end-expiratory pressure (PEEP).

Monitoring: Continuous monitoring of ventilator settings, arterial blood gases, and respiratory mechanics is essential to adjust ventilation parameters and manage complications.

9. *Complications and monitoring:*
   Complications: Monitoring for complications such as ventilator-associated pneumonia, barotrauma, and cardiovascular instability is crucial.
   Serial assessments: Serial clinical assessments, chest X-rays, and laboratory tests guide ongoing management and response to treatment.
   In summary, ventilation strategies focus on improving oxygenation, reducing the work of breathing, and managing fluid status while addressing the underlying cause. The choice between noninvasive and invasive ventilation depends on the severity of respiratory distress and response to initial interventions.
   The treatment of pulmonary edema in preeclampsia is similar to those of nonpregnant patients and includes oxygen therapy, fluid restriction, intravenous furosemide (80 mg initially), and central hemodynamic monitoring. Reduction in afterload is obtained with the use of vasodilators (hydralazine, nifedipine). Noninvasive ventilation should be tried as the initial technique before tracheal intubation. Decrease of critically high blood pressure using an intravenous antihypertensive is also necessary. Nitroglycerin (glyceryl trinitrate) is recommended for the management of a pregnant woman with acute pulmonary edema. Other alternative agents are: sodium nitroprusside, intravenous furosemide, calcium channel antagonists such as nicardipine or nifedipine, prazosin as well as hydralazine may also be considered.

Q7. What is the obstetric management in antenatal patients with pulmonary edema?

Managing an antenatal patient with pulmonary edema requires prompt recognition, appropriate interventions, and close monitoring to ensure maternal and fetal well-being. The occurrence of pulmonary edema indicates the urgent termination of pregnancy.

Fetal monitoring: Monitor fetal well-being with continuous fetal heart rate monitoring and periodic assessment of fetal movements.

Timing: Depending on the severity of the pulmonary edema and preeclampsia, delivery may be indicated to resolve the condition definitively.

Mode of delivery: The mode of delivery (vaginal vs. cesarean) depends on maternal and fetal status, gestational age, and obstetric indications.

Psychological support: Emotional support and reassurance to alleviate anxiety and promote patient cooperation with treatment is very important.

Postpartum monitoring: Monitoring of maternal and neonatal status closely postpartum is important as some complications can persist or develop after delivery.

Pulmonary edema could be a factor influencing the decision for pregnancy termination. The American Congress of Obstetricians and Gynecologists strongly recommends delivery irrespective of gestational age for preeclamptic women whose condition is complicated with pulmonary edema.

NPPV can be administered safely to pregnant women with preeclampsia-induced pulmonary edema. The decision to intubate or terminate the pregnancy should be made without delay when the maternal or fetal condition worsens. Delivery must be expedited to avert poor perinatal and maternal outcomes.

In summary, managing an antenatal patient with pulmonary edema requires a systematic approach focusing on stabilization, addressing underlying causes such as preeclampsia, optimizing fluid balance, and ensuring appropriate pharmacological interventions while closely monitoring maternal and fetal well-being. Collaboration among healthcare providers and timely intervention is crucial to achieving optimal outcomes for both the mother and the baby.

Q8. What are the long-term implications, when pulmonary edema occurs with preeclampsia?

Long-term implications of pulmonary edema, especially in the context of conditions like preeclampsia, can vary depending on several factors, including the severity of the initial episode, the underlying health of the individual, and promptness of treatment. Potential long-term implications include:

Respiratory function: Severe pulmonary edema can lead to lung injury and impairments in gas exchange. While acute pulmonary edema can often be managed effectively with appropriate treatment, recurrent or severe episodes may contribute to chronic respiratory issues such as decreased lung function, chronic cough, or exercise intolerance.

Cardiovascular health: Preeclampsia itself is associated with cardiovascular risks in the long term, including hypertension and increased risk of cardiovascular disease later in life. Pulmonary edema, particularly if severe, can strain the heart and contribute to long-term cardiac dysfunction or structural changes.

Renal function: Preeclampsia and severe pulmonary edema can affect renal function acutely. Although most cases resolve with treatment, there is a risk of long-term kidney damage or chronic kidney disease, especially in cases of severe or recurrent preeclampsia.

Psychological impact: Experiencing severe medical complications during pregnancy, such as pulmonary edema, can have lasting psychological effects. This may include anxiety related to future pregnancies or concerns about long-term health consequences.

Risk of recurrence: Women who have experienced preeclampsia with pulmonary edema have a higher risk of recurrence in subsequent pregnancies. Proper preconception counseling and management are crucial to mitigate these risks.

Quality of life: Chronic symptoms or disabilities resulting from severe pulmonary edema can impact the overall quality of life, affecting daily activities, employment, and social interactions.

Follow-up and monitoring: Individuals who have experienced pulmonary edema during pregnancy, especially in the context of preeclampsia, require long-term follow-up to monitor cardiovascular and renal health. Regular assessments may include blood pressure monitoring, echocardiography, and renal function tests.

In summary, while many cases of pulmonary edema related to preeclampsia can be successfully managed with appropriate medical intervention, there can be long-term implications for respiratory, cardiovascular, and renal health. Close monitoring, timely intervention, and ongoing medical follow-up are essential to minimize these risks and optimize long-term outcomes.

Q9. What preventive measures can be taken to avoid this complication?

Preventive measures for pulmonary edema, particularly in the context of conditions like preeclampsia, focus on managing risk factors and early recognition of signs and symptoms to prevent progression to severe complications.

Antenatal care: Regular prenatal visits and early detection of preeclampsia risk factors (such as hypertension, proteinuria, and edema) are crucial. Monitoring blood pressure and urine protein levels at each visit helps identify preeclampsia early.

Blood pressure management: Effective management of hypertension during pregnancy is essential. This may involve lifestyle modifications, medication as prescribed by a healthcare provider, and close monitoring of blood pressure levels.

Monitoring fluid status: Monitoring fluid intake and output can help prevent fluid overload, which is a contributing factor to pulmonary edema. Healthcare providers should assess for signs of fluid retention, such as rapid weight gain, edema (especially in the lower extremities), and difficulty breathing.

Early recognition of symptoms: Educating pregnant individuals about the signs and symptoms of preeclampsia and pulmonary edema (such as severe headache, visual disturbances, sudden weight gain, swelling, and shortness of breath) promotes early recognition and timely medical intervention.

Lifestyle modifications: Encouraging a healthy lifestyle, including regular physical activity as recommended by a healthcare provider, maintaining a balanced diet, and avoiding excessive salt intake, can help manage blood pressure and reduce the risk of preeclampsia.

Medication compliance: Compliance with prescribed medications, such as antihypertensive drugs or medications to prevent seizures in severe cases of preeclampsia (eclampsia), is crucial to manage the condition and reduce the risk of complications like pulmonary edema.

Timely medical intervention: Prompt medical evaluation and management of preeclampsia are essential to prevent its progression to severe forms that can lead to pulmonary edema and other complications.

Delivery planning: In cases where preeclampsia cannot be controlled or when complications arise, timely delivery of the baby and placenta may be necessary to resolve the condition and prevent further complications, including pulmonary edema.

In summary, preventive measures for pulmonary edema in the context of preeclampsia focus on early detection, effective management of blood pressure and fluid status, lifestyle modifications, patient education, and timely medical intervention when necessary. These measures aim to optimize maternal and fetal outcomes during pregnancy and reduce the risk of serious complications.

BIBLIOGRAPHY

1. Abildgaard U, Heimdal K. Pathogenesis of the syndrome of hemolysis, elevated liver enzymes, and low platelet count (HELLP): a review. Eur J Obstet Gynecol Reprod Biol. 2013;166(2):117-23.
2. Alexander JM. Clinical management. In: Taylor RN (Eds). Chesley's Hypertensive Disorders in Pregnancy, 5th edition. Philadelphia: Elsevier; 2015. pp. 439-64.
3. Alonso-Ventura V, Li Y, Pasupuleti V, et al. Effects of preeclampsia and eclampsia on maternal metabolic and biochemical outcomes in later life: a systematic review and meta-analysis. Metabolism. 2020;102:154012.
4. American College of Obstetricians and Gynaecologists. Hypertension in pregnancy. Report of the American College of Obstetricians and Gynecologists' Task Force on Hypertension in Pregnancy. Obstet Gynecol. 2013;122(5):1122-31.
5. American College of Obstetricians and Gynecologists. ACOG Practice Bulletin No. 203: chronic hypertension in pregnancy. Obstet Gynecol. 2019;133(1):e26-50.
6. American College of Obstetricians and Gynecologists. ACOG Practice Bulletin No. 207: thrombocytopenia in pregnancy. Obstet Gynecol. 2019;133(3):e181-93.

7. American College of Obstetricians and Gynecologists. ACOG Practice Bulletin No. 107: induction of labor. Obstet Gynecol. 2009;114(2 Pt 1):386-97.
8. American College of Obstetricians and Gynecologists. Gestational Hypertension and Preeclampsia: ACOG Practice Bulletin: Number 222. Obstet Gynecol. 2020;135:e237-60.
9. Assaad S, Kratzert WB, Shelley B, et al. Assessment of Pulmonary Edema: Principles and Practice. J Cardiothorac Vasc Anesth. 2018;32(2):901-14.
10. Audibert F, Friedman SA, Frangieh AY, et al. Clinical utility of strict diagnostic criteria for the HELLP (hemolysis, elevated liver enzymes, and low platelets) syndrome. Am J Obstet Gynecol. 1996;175(2):460-4.
11. Bacal CJO, Maina JW, Nandurkar HH, et al. Blood apheresis technologies: a critical review on challenges towards efficient blood separation and treatment. Materials Advances. 2021;2(22):7210-36.
12. Baskaran J, Lopez RA, Cassagnol M. (2024). Prothrombin complex concentrate. [online] Available from https://www.ncbi.nlm.nih.gov/books/NBK539716/. [Last accessed November, 2024]
13. Bhorat I, Naidoo DP, Moodley J. Maternal cardiac hemodynamics in severe pre-eclampsia complicated by acute pulmonary edema: a review. J Matern Fetal Neonatal Med. 2016;30(23):2769-77.
14. Brandt JS, Ananth CV. Placental abruption at near-term and term gestations: pathophysiology, epidemiology, diagnosis, and management. Am J Obstet Gynecol. 2023;228(5S):S1313-29.
15. Casella J, Perry M. (2024). EMS Tactical Paramedic Lethal Triad. [online] Available from https://www.ncbi.nlm.nih.gov/books/NBK603758/. [Last accessed November, 2024]
16. Cavaignac-Vitalis M, Vidal F, Simon-Toulza C, et al. Conservative versus active management in HELLP syndrome: results from a cohort study. J Matern Fetal Neonatal Med. 2019;32(11):1769-75.
17. Chawla N, Shah H, Huynh K, et al. The role of platelet-activating factor and magnesium in obstetrics and gynecology: is there crosstalk between pre-eclampsia, clinical hypertension, and HELLP syndrome? Biomedicines. 2023;11(5):1343.
18. Churchill D, Duley L, Thornton JG, et al. Interventionist versus expectant care for severe pre-eclampsia between 24 and 34 weeks gestation. Cochrane Database Syst Rev. 2018;10(10):CD003106.
19. Committee on Obstetric Practice. Committee Opinion No. 692: emergent therapy for acute-onset, severe hypertension during pregnancy and the postpartum period. Obstet Gynecol. 2017;129(4):e90-5.
20. Costello RA, Nehring SM. (2024). Disseminated intravascular coagulation. [online] Available from https://www.ncbi.nlm.nih.gov/books/NBK441834/. [Last accessed November, 2024]
21. Cunningham FG, Nelson DB. Disseminated intravascular coagulation syndromes in obstetrics. Obstet Gynecol. 2015;126(5):999-1011.
22. Dennis AT, Solnordal CB. Acute pulmonary edema in pregnant women. Anesthesia. 2012;67(6):646-59.
23. Erez O, Othman M, Rabinovich A, et al. DIC in pregnancy–pathophysiology, clinical characteristics, diagnostic scores, and treatments. J Blood Med. 2022;13:21-44.

24. Fishel Bartal M, Sibai BM. Eclampsia in the 21st century. Am J Obstet Gynecol. 2022;226(2S):S1237-53.
25. Fitzpatrick KE, Hinshaw K, Kurinczuk JJ, et al. Risk factors, management, and outcomes of hemolysis, elevated liver enzymes, and low platelets syndrome and elevated liver enzymes, low platelets syndrome. Obstet Gynecol. 2014;123(3):618-27.
26. Fonseca JE, Otero JC, Messa C. Dexamethasone for the treatment of class I HELLP syndrome: a double-blind, placebo-controlled, multicenter, randomized clinical trial. Pregnancy Hypertens. 2019;17:158-64.
27. Gandhi S, Sun D, Park AL, et al. The Pulmonary Edema Preeclampsia Evaluation (PEPE) Study. J Obstet Gynaecol Can. 2014;36:1065-70.
28. Govil D, Pal D. Point-of-care testing of coagulation in intensive care unit: role of thromboelastography. Indian J Crit Care Med. 2019;23(Suppl 3):S202-6.
29. Haram K, Mortensen JH, Nagy B. Genetic aspects of preeclampsia and the HELLP syndrome. J Pregnancy. 2014;2014:910751.
30. Haram K, Svendsen E, Abildgaard U. The HELLP syndrome: clinical issues and management. A review. BMC Pregnancy Childbirth. 2009;9:8.
31. Jayawardena L, Mcnamara E. Diagnosis and management of pregnancies complicated by haemolysis, elevated liver enzymes and low platelets (HELLP) syndrome in the tertiary setting. Intern Med J. 2020;50(3):342-9.
32. Johnson JD, Louis JM. Does race or ethnicity play a role in the origin, pathophysiology, and outcomes of preeclampsia? An expert review of the literature. Am J Obstet Gynecol. 2022;226(2S):S876-85.
33. Kadikar SK, Divan FJ, Topiwala U, et al. Study of pregnancy with disseminated intravascular coagulation. Int J Reprod Contrac Obstet Gynecol. 2021;10(11):4220-6.
34. Kaur H, Kolli M. Acute pulmonary edema in pregnancy - fluid overload or atypical pre-eclampsia. Cureus. 2021;13(11):e19305.
35. Khayat S, Ali M, Almasoudi L, et al. The Impact of BiLevel Positive Airway Pressure (BiPAP) Application Timing on Emergency Room Length of Stay in Patients with Pulmonary Edema: A Single-Center, Retrospective Cohort Study. Cureus. 2022;14(12):e33193.
36. Lachmeijer AM, Arngrímsson R, Bastiaans EJ, et al. A genome-wide scan for preeclampsia in the Netherlands. Eur J Hum Genet. 2001;9(10):758-64.
37. Leeman L, Dresang LT, Fontaine P. Hypertensive disorders of pregnancy. Am Fam Physician. 2016;93(2):121-7.
38. Magee LA, Brown MA, Hall DR, et al. The 2021 International Society for the Study of Hypertension in Pregnancy classification, diagnosis & management recommendations for international practice. Pregnancy Hypertens. 2022;27: 148-69.
39. Magee LA, Pels A, Helewa M, et al. Diagnosis, evaluation, and management of the hypertensive disorders of pregnancy. Pregnancy Hypertens. 2014;4(2):105-45.
40. Magee LA, Smith GN, Bloch C, et al. Guideline no. 426: hypertensive disorders of pregnancy: diagnosis, prediction, prevention, and management. J Obstet Gynaecol Can. 2022;44(5):547-71.e1.
41. Malek R, Soufi S. (2023). Pulmonary Edema. [online] Available from https://www.ncbi.nlm.nih.gov/books/NBK557611/. [Last accessed November, 2024]

42. Millogo T, Sawadogo S Nee M, et al. Lupus anticoagulant and severe pre-eclampsia or eclampsia: a hospital-based case-control study in Ouagadougou, Burkina Faso. Int J Med Lab Res. 2021;6(3):1-5.
43. Minakami H, Morikawa M, Yamada T, et al. Differentiation of acute fatty liver of pregnancy from syndrome of hemolysis, elevated liver enzymes and low platelet counts. J Obstet Gynaecol Res. 2014;40(3):641-9.
44. Ness PM, Campbell-Lee SA. Single donor versus pooled random donor platelet concentrates. Curr Opin Hematol. 2001;8(6):392-6.
45. Ngene NC, Moodley J. Blood pressure measurement and rapid-acting antihypertensives for severe hypertension in pregnancy. Obstet Gynaecol Forum. 2016;26(3):35-40.
46. Padden MO. HELLP syndrome: recognition and perinatal management. Am Fam Physician. 1999;60(3):829-36.
47. Parker SE, Werler MM, Gissler M, et al. Placental abruption and subsequent risk of pre-eclampsia: a population-based case-control study. Paediatr Perinat Epidemiol. 2015;29(3):211-9.
48. Poimenidi E, Metodiev Y, Archer NN, et al. Haemolysis, elevated liver enzymes and low platelets: diagnosis and management in critical care. J Intensive Care Soc. 2022;23(3):372-8.
49. Ramos JGL, Sass N, Costa SHM. Preeclampsia. Rev Bras Ginecol Obstet. 2017;39(9):496-512.
50. Rao D, Chaudhari NK, Moore RM, et al. HELLP syndrome: a diagnostic conundrum with severe complications. BMJ Case Rep. 2016;2016:bcr2016216802.
51. Rattray DD, O'Connell CM, Baskett TF. Acute disseminated intravascular coagulation in obstetrics: a tertiary centre population review (1980 to 2009). J Obstet Gynaecol Canada. 2012;34(4):341-7.
52. Robertson L, Wu O, Langhorne P, et al. Thrombophilia in pregnancy: a systematic review. Br J Haematol. 2006;132(2):171-96.
53. Schmid S, Friesenecker B, Lorenz I, et al. Administration of recombinant activated factor VII (NovoSeven) in three cases of uncontrolled bleeding caused by disseminated intravascular coagulopathy. Clin Appl Thromb Hemost. 2007;13(3):313-7.
54. Seckin NC, Inegöl I, Turhan NÖ, et al. A life-threatening second trimester disseminated intravascular coagulopathy with protein S deficiency. Clin Appl Thromb Hemost. 2004;10(3):289-91.
55. Sibai BM. Diagnosis, controversies, and management of the syndrome of hemolysis, elevated liver enzymes, and low platelet count. Obstet Gynecol. 2004;103(5 Pt 1):981-91.
56. Soma-Pillay P, Nelson-Piercy C, Tolppanen H, et al. Physiological changes in pregnancy. Cardiovasc J Afr. 2016;27:89-94.
57. Sriram S, Robertson MS. Critically ill obstetric patients in Australia: a retrospective audit of 8 years′ experience in a tertiary intensive care unit. Crit Care Resusc. 2008;10(2):124.
58. Thornton CE, von Dadelszen P, Makris A, et al. Acute Pulmonary Oedema as a Complication of Hypertension During Pregnancy. Hypertens Pregnancy. 2009;30(2):169-79.

59. Tikkanen M. Placental abruption: epidemiology, risk factors and consequences. Acta Obstetricia et Gynecologica Scandinavica. 2011;90:140-9.
60. Turgut A, Demirci O, Demirci E, et al. Comparison of maternal and neonatal outcomes in women with HELLP syndrome and women with severe preeclampsia without HELLP syndrome. J Prenat Med. 2010;4(3):51-8.
61. Ulvin LB, Heuser K, Olsen KB, et al. Factors associated with refractoriness and outcome in an adult status epilepticus cohort. Seizure. 2018;61:111-8.
62. Varlas VN, Bohîlțea R, Gheorghe G, et al. State of the art in hepatic dysfunction in pregnancy. Healthcare (Basel). 2021;9(11):1481.
63. Woudstra DM, Chandra S, Hofmeyr GJ, et al. Corticosteroids for HELLP (hemolysis, elevated liver enzymes, low platelets) syndrome in pregnancy. Cochrane Database Syst Rev. 2010;(9):CD008148.

CHAPTER 13

Anesthesia in Preeclampsia

Hemant Mehta

PREANESTHESIA EVALUATION

- Patients with preeclampsia should be assessed by the anesthesia team early in the peripartum period, with the higher chance for the need of emergency delivery during the course of pregnancy. The patient should be assessed with special focus on the airway, hemodynamic status, and coagulation abnormalities.
- Preeclamptic patients are often at risk for airway edema. During labor and delivery, the airway edema may worsen leading to challenges in airway management.
- Thrombocytopenia and other coagulopathies may occur in severe preeclampsia, hence neuraxial anesthesia techniques may be contraindicated because of the risk of spinal epidural hematoma.
- Epidural catheters are to be placed early in labor in patients with declining platelet counts. Epidural catheters can be placed for patients with a platelet count >70,000/μL, and no to be used if the platelet count is ≤50,000/μL, and to be used depending upon risk versus benefit in an individual case with a platelet count between 50,000 and 70,000/μL.

INTRAVENOUS FLUID AND BLOOD PRESSURE MANAGEMENT

- Infusion of intravenous (IV) fluids should be restricted for patients with preeclampsia to in order to prevent pulmonary edema due to fluid overload. Fluid bolus is not recommended for initiation of labor analgesia, and preloading with fluid prior to neuraxial anesthesia for cesarean delivery should be avoided or limited to <500 mL.
- Blood pressure targets are to be preferably maintained as close to the patient's baseline and should never exceed systolic >160 mm Hg and diastolic >110 mm Hg.
- Antihypertensive agents that can be used with reasonable efficacy and safety in pregnancy to manage hypertension are labetalol, nifedipine, and hydralazine.
- Only very small doses of vasopressors should be used if at all (e.g., ephedrine 2.5–5 mg IV, phenylephrine 25–50 μg IV).

Flowchart 1: Decision making for providing neuraxial anesthesia in obstetric patients with thrombocytopenia.

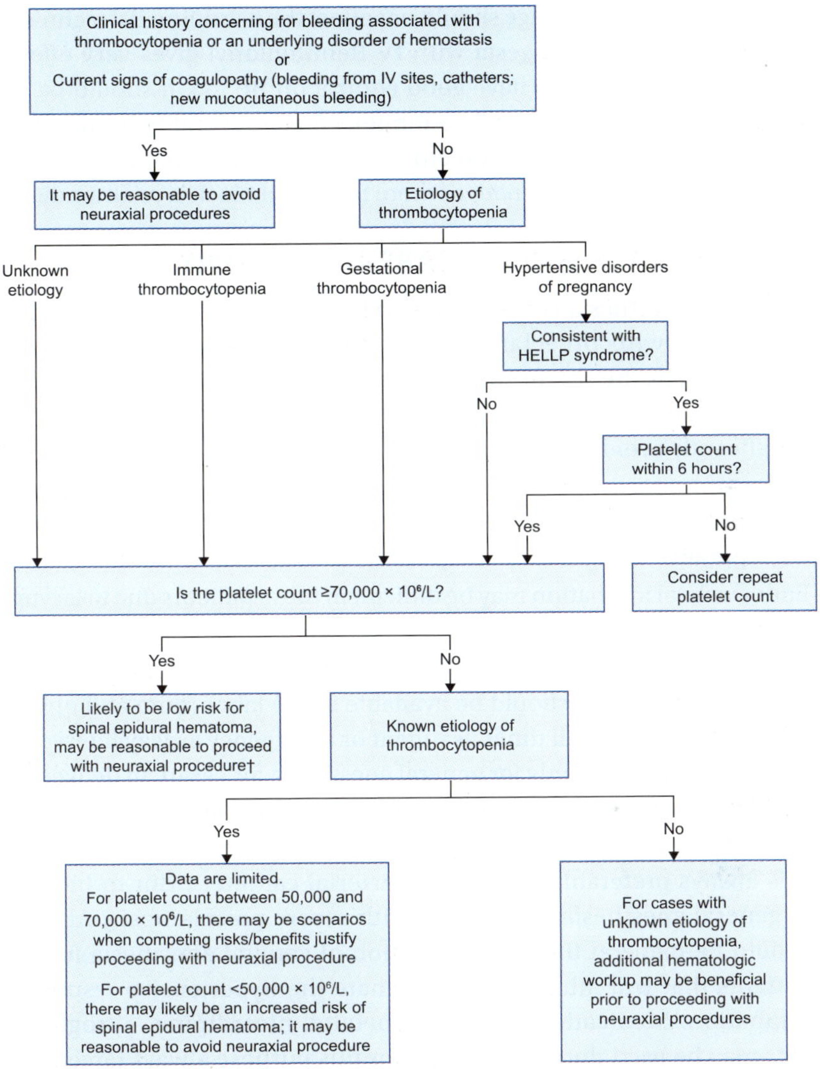

PAIN RELIEF DURING LABOR

- Neuraxial analgesia can be used for providing labor analgesia in patients with preeclampsia.
- Continuous neuraxial analgesia is to known to lessen the hypertensive response to intrapartum pain and circulating catecholamines, and additionally is beneficial for conversion to surgical neuraxial anesthesia quickly and avoidance of general anesthesia.

- The American College of Obstetricians and Gynecologists recommends use of low-dose aspirin for prevention of preeclampsia in high-risk patients, however its usage should not affect the use neuraxial techniques.
- Patient controlled analgesia with IV Remifentanyl gives very effective pain relief and helps to have good control on BP too. It should be used with lots of care, caution and continuous maternal and fetus monitoring with 1:1 care. Remifentanyl do cross-placental barrier but it is very short acting and it is good alternative where neuraxial block is contraindicated.

ANESTHESIA DURING CESAREAN DELIVERY

- Neuraxial anesthesia is always preferable rather than general anesthesia in patients with preeclampsia in whom cesarean delivery is to be performed, as the risk of severe hypertension which may turn out to be life threatening during induction of anesthesia or during emergency is significantly avoided.
- Neuraxial anesthesia using intrathecal/epidural buprenorphine not only helps managing patient intraoperatively but it give profound postoperative analgesia and helps to keep vitals in normal limit.
- Endotracheal intubation may be difficult in these patients due to laryngeal edema.
- The necessary equipment needed to manage difficult and emergency airway management should be available in the labor room and obstetric operation theater at all times as urgent or emergency airway intervention may be required not only for general anesthesia for cesarean delivery, but also for airway protection if eclamptic seizures occur, or in the setting of magnesium toxicity.
- It is always preferable to insert an arterial catheter prior to induction of general anesthesia for patients with severe preeclampsia. All efforts should be made at the tie of induction of general anesthesia for these patients that will minimize or eliminate the hypertensive response to intubation. Medications such as labetalol, nicardipine, nitroglycerin, etc., may be used during induction for this purpose always targeting the systolic blood pressure to <160 mm Hg.
- While on the other hand spinal, epidural, and combined spinal-epidural anesthesia are certainly safer.
- To avoid the occurrence of neuraxial anesthesia-induced hypotension for patients with preeclampsia, titrated low-dose phenylephrine (i.e., starting at <50 μg/min) or phenylephrine rescue boluses (e.g., 25–50 μg IV) may be infused.
- If bradycardia is present then ephedrine (5–10 mg IV bolus, or 1–5 mg/min IV infusion) should be used instead.

INDUCTION OF GENERAL ANESTHESIA

The following steps are generally to be followed during induction of anesthesia:

- Preinduction, labetalol 10 mg IV boluses, titrated to achieve systolic blood pressure <160 mm Hg, if time permits.
- Propofol 2 mg/kg IV
- Succinylcholine 1 mg/kg IV
- Nitroglycerin infusion, or nicardipine (100 μg/mL, 1–2 mL bolus), as needed during induction, with goal systolic blood pressure <160 mm Hg.
- In order to blunt the hypertensive response to intubation the following medications may be used:
    - Labetalol titrated with 10 mg IV boluses up to 1 mg/kg prior to induction
    - Esmolol 2 mg/kg IV during induction, or 1 mg/kg IV with lidocaine
    - Nitroglycerin 1.5–2.5 μg/kg IV
    - Nicardipine 15–30 μg/kg IV, or 100–200 μg bolus during induction
    - Fentanyl 1–3 μg/kg IV
    - Remifentanil 1 μg/kg IV during induction, crosses the placenta and may cause transient neonatal respiratory depression.
- Opioids are generally avoided during induction of anesthesia for cesarean delivery due to concerns for neonatal respiratory depression.
- Neonatology team should be aware of all medications administered to the mother during induction of general anesthesia.

MAGNESIUM THERAPY

- Magnesium sulfate is the anticonvulsant of choice to both prevent and treat eclamptic seizures in severely preeclamptic patients and should be routinely administered as per the standard regimen even in the operating room during cesarean delivery.
- Magnesium does not potentiate the effects of succinylcholine, and the usual rapid sequence induction dose (i.e., succinylcholine 1–1.5 mg/kg IV) should be administered.
- When muscle relaxation is required, a small additional dose of succinylcholine (10–20 mg IV) or deeper anesthesia may be sufficient.
- Potentiation of the effects of nondepolarizing neuromuscular blocking agents (NMBAs) is known to occur in patients receiving magnesium sulfate which can prolong the duration of action of rocuronium, cisatracurium, and vecuronium.

  Since nondepolarizing NMBAs are rarely necessary during cesarean delivery, they should be avoided for patients who are receiving magnesium.

- If a longer duration of muscle relaxation is necessary, to allow for better surgical conditions prior to or during fascial closure, small incremental doses of non-depolarizing NMBA (i.e., rocuronium 10–20 mg IV or cisatracurium 2–4 mg IV) should be administered, and titrated to effect using a twitch monitor with the goal of one twitch in the train of four twitches.
- Quantitative or qualitative monitoring should also be used at the end of surgery to ensure adequate reversal of neuromuscular blockade.

UTEROTONIC MEDICATIONS

- Uterotonics to be administered after delivery of the fetus during both vaginal and cesarean delivery.
- Oxytocin is the first line medication, followed by other uterotonics if bleeding persists. The oxytocin dose generally is to be increased in preeclamptic patients who receive magnesium sulfate infusions.
- Methylergometrine can cause severe hypertension, and should not be administered to patients with preeclampsia.
- For postpartum hemorrhage unresponsive to oxytocin administration, prostaglandins (i.e., misoprostol or carboprost) should be administered. Carboprost should be avoided in patients with asthma.

POSTOPERATIVE PAIN CONTROL

- NSAIDs are opioid sparing, and are especially effective for relief of uterine cramping, though these medications interfere with platelet function.
- Practice Bulletin from the American Congress of Obstetricians and Gynecologists (ACOG) 2020 recommends the use of NSAIDS preferentially over opioids for postpartum pain in patients with hypertensive disorders, including preeclampsia.
- Epidural buprenorphine not only helps managing patient intraoperatively but it give profound postoperative analgesia and helps to keep vitals in normal limit.
- For patients who undergo cesarean delivery, need for postoperative monitoring in the post anesthesia recovery unit or intensive care unit is based on the intraoperative course, patient factors, the need for ongoing invasive monitoring, and available resources.

BIBLIOGRAPHY

1. ACOG.org. (2021). American College of Obstetricians and Gynecologists' Practice Advisory: Low-Dose Aspirin Use for the Prevention of Preeclampsia and Related Morbidity and Mortality. [online] Available from https://www.acog.org/clinical/clinical-guidance/practice-advisory/articles/2021/12/

low-dose-aspirin-use-for-the-prevention-of-preeclampsia-and-related-morbidity-and-mortality [Last accessed November, 2024].

2. Acog.org. (2021). Hypertension in Pregnancy. [online] Available from http://www.acog.org/Resources-And-Publications/Task-Force-and-Work-Group-Reports/Hypertension-in-Pregnancy. [Last accessed November, 2024].
3. American College of Obstetricians and Gynecologists. Gestational Hypertension and Preeclampsia: ACOG Practice Bulletin: Number 222. Obstet Gynecol. 2020;135:e237-60.
4. Aya AG, Vialles N, Tanoubi I, et al. Spinal anesthesia-induced hypotension: a risk comparison between patients with severe preeclampsia and healthy women undergoing preterm cesarean delivery. Anesth Analg. 2005;101:869.
5. Bauer ME, Arendt K, Beilin Y, et al. The Society for Obstetric Anesthesia and Perinatology Interdisciplinary Consensus Statement on Neuraxial Procedures in Obstetric Patients with Thrombocytopenia. Anesth Analg. 2021;132:1531.
6. Committee on Obstetric Practice. Committee Opinion No. 692: emergent therapy for acute-onset, severe hypertension during pregnancy and the postpartum period. Obstet Gynecol. 2017;129(4):e90-5.
7. Duley L, Williams J, Henderson-Smart DJ. Plasma volume expansion for treatment of women with pre-eclampsia. Cochrane Database Syst Rev. 2000;1999(4):CD001805.
8. Dyer RA, Els I, Farbas J, et al. Prospective, randomized trial comparing general with spinal anesthesia for cesarean delivery in preeclamptic patients with a nonreassuring fetal heart trace. Anesthesiology. 2003;99:561.
9. Head BB, Owen J, Vincent RD Jr, et al. A randomized trial of intrapartum analgesia in women with severe preeclampsia. Obstet Gynecol. 2002;99:452.
10. Hofmeyr G, Cyna A, Middleton P. Prophylactic intravenous preloading for regional analgesia in labour. Cochrane Database Syst Rev. 2004:CD000175.
11. Loubert C. Fluid and vasopressor management for Cesarean delivery under spinal anesthesia: continuing professional development. Can J Anaesth. 2012;59:604.
12. Mohta M, Duggal S, Chilkoti GT. Randomised double-blind comparison of bolus phenylephrine or ephedrine for treatment of hypotension in women with pre-eclampsia undergoing caesarean section. Anaesthesia. 2018;73:839.
13. Nice.org.uk. (2011). Hypertension in pregnancy. The management of hypertensive disorders during pregnancy. London (UK): National Institute for Health and Clinical Excellence (NICE); (Clinical guideline; no. 107). [online] Available from https://www.nice.org.uk/guidance/cg107 [Last accessed November, 2024].
14. Pant M, Fong R, Scavone B. Prevention of peri-induction hypertension in preeclamptic patients: a focused review. Anesth Analg. 2014;119:1350.
15. Podovei M, Bateman BT. The Consensus Bundle on Hypertension in Pregnancy and the Anesthesiologist: Doing All the Right Things for All the Patients All of the Time. Anesth Analg. 2017;125:383.
16. Pretorius T, van Rensburg G, Dyer RA, et al. The influence of fluid management on outcomes in preeclampsia: a systematic review and meta-analysis. Int J Obstet Anesth. 2018;34:85.

17. Regitz-Zagrosek V, Roos-Hesselink JW, Bauersachs J, et al. 2018 ESC Guidelines for the management of cardiovascular diseases during pregnancy. Eur Heart J 2018; 39:3165.
18. Tyagi A, Mohan A, Singh Y, et al. Effective Dose of Prophylactic Oxytocin Infusion During Cesarean Delivery in 90% Population of Nonlaboring Patients with Preeclampsia Receiving Magnesium Sulfate Therapy and Normotensives: An Up-Down Sequential Allocation Dose-Response Study. Anesth Analg. 2022;134:303.
19. Visalyaputra S, Rodanant O, Somboonviboon W, et al. Spinal versus epidural anesthesia for cesarean delivery in severe preeclampsia: a prospective randomized, multicenter study. Anesth Analg. 2005;101:862.